Student Activity Guide

Guide to Good Food

Deborah L. Bence, CFCS
*Family and Consumer Science
    Author and Editor
Homewood, Illinois*

Claudia A. Lazok
*Curriculum Specialist,
    Tucson Unified School District
Tuscon, Arizona*

Guide to Good Food Text
    *by Velda L. Largen
    and Deborah L. Bence, CFCS*

Publisher
The Goodheart-Willcox Company, Inc.
Tinley Park, Illinois

Introduction

This *Student Activity Guide* is designed for use with the text *Guide to Good Food*. It will help you understand and remember the facts and concepts about food and nutrition presented in the text. It will also help you apply this learning in your daily life.

The activities in this guide are divided into chapters that correspond to the chapters in the text. By reading the text first, you will have the information you need to complete the activities. Try to complete the activities without referring to the text. If necessary, you can look at the book again later to complete any questions you could not answer. At that time, you can also compare the answers you have to the information in the book.

You will find a number of types of activities in this guide. Many of the activities, such as crossword puzzles, word mazes, true and false questions, and fill-in-the-blank sentences, have "right" answers. These activities can be used as review guides when you study for tests and quizzes. Other activities, such as evaluations and comparisons, will ask for opinions and ideas that cannot be judged as "right" or "wrong." These activities are designed to stimulate your thinking and help you apply information presented in the text.

The activities in this guide have been designed to increase your interest and understanding of the text material. The more thought you put into the activities, the more knowledge you will gain from them.

Copyright 1996

by

The Goodheart-Willcox Company, Inc.

Previous Editions Copyright 1992, 1988, 1984, 1982

International Standard Book Number 1-56637-246-1

2 3 4 5 6 7 8 9 10 96 00 99 98 97 96

Contents

How Food Affects Life

Your Food Habits

Activity A

Chapter 1

Name_____

Date_____ Period_____

Answer the following questions about your food habits.

1. How many meals do you eat each day? _____

2. How many snacks do you eat each day? _____

3. What size portions do you eat?_____

4. How often do you take second helpings?_____

5. How much time do you spend at each meal? _____

6. What times of day do you eat? _____

7. Is your eating behavior different on weekends than it is on weekdays? If so, explain why. _____

_____

8. Where do you do most of your eating?_____

9. With whom do you do most of your eating? _____

10. What factors, other than hunger, sometimes cause you to eat?_____

_____

11. What else, if anything, do you do while you are eating?_____

12. How does food make you feel? _____

13. What do you grab to satisfy hunger in a hurry? _____

14. What is your favorite food?_____

15. Name a food you do not like and explain why you do not like it._____

_____

16. How does culture affect your food habits?_____

_____

17. How does your lifestyle affect your food habits? _____

_____

18. How do family members and friends affect your food habits?_____

_____

19. How does mass media affect your food habits? _____

_____

20. How do current trends affect your food habits? _____

_____

Advertising Analysis

Activity B   Name_____

Chapter 1   Date _____ Period _____

Clip an advertisement for a food product from a newspaper or magazine and mount it in the space below. Then answer the questions that follow.

1. Is this a new food product or one that has been available for some time? _____

   _____

2. Describe the technique(s) used to encourage you to buy this product._____

   _____

   _____

   _____

3. What useful information does this advertisement give you about the product?_____

   _____

   _____

   _____

4. After seeing this advertisement, would you be interested in using this product? Explain why or why not.

   _____

   _____

Nutritional Needs

Nutrient Facts

Activity A

Chapter 2

Name_____

Date _____ Period _____

After researching or discussing the various nutrients, list their function(s) and food sources in the chart. Then answer the questions that follow.

Nutrient	Function(s)	Food Sources
Carbohydrates		
Fats		
Proteins		
Vitamin A		
Vitamin D		
Vitamin E		
Vitamin K		
Vitamin C (Ascorbic acid)		
Thiamin (Vitamin B-1)		
Riboflavin (Vitamin B-2)		
Niacin		
Vitamin B-6 (Pyridoxine)		
Folic acid		
Vitamin B-12		

(Continued)

Name _____

Nutrient	Function(s)	Food Sources
Pantothenic acid		
Biotin		
Calcium		
Phosphorus		
Magnesium		
Sodium Chlorine Potassium		
Iron		
Iodine		
Manganese		
Copper		
Zinc		
Fluorine		
Water		

1. Do you regularly eat sources of each of the nutrients listed in this chart? _____

2. If you answered no to the above question, which nutrients are lacking in your diet? _____

    _____

3. Why is it necessary to include sources of each of these nutrients in your diet?_____

    _____

    _____

4. How can this chart serve as a guide in choosing the foods you eat? _____

    _____

    _____

5. How would you define good nutrition? _____

    _____

Nutrient Deficiencies and Excesses

Activity B   Name _____

Chapter 2   Date _____ Period _____

Match the following nutrient deficiencies and excesses on the left with the descriptions of their symptoms on the right. Beneath each item, check the minus (–) box if the condition is caused by a nutrient deficiency. Check the plus (+) box if the condition is caused by a nutrient excess. Then write the name of the nutrient related to the condition in the blank.

_____ 1. dental caries

– ☐ + ☐   _____

_____ 2. atherosclerosis

– ☐ + ☐   _____

_____ 3. kwashiorkor

– ☐ + ☐   _____

_____ 4. night blindness

– ☐ + ☐   _____

_____ 5. rickets

– ☐ + ☐   _____

_____ 6. scurvy

– ☐ + ☐   _____

_____ 7. beriberi

– ☐ + ☐   _____

_____ 8. pellagra

– ☐ + ☐   _____

_____ 9. pernicious anemia

– ☐ + ☐   _____

_____ 10. osteoporosis

– ☐ + ☐   _____

_____ 11. edema

– ☐ + ☐   _____

_____ 12. anemia

– ☐ + ☐   _____

_____ 13. endemic goiter

– ☐ + ☐   _____

A. numbness in ankles and legs followed by severe cramping and subsequent paralysis

B. inability to see in the dark

C. enlargement of the thyroid gland

D. loss of appetite, pale skin, and tiredness

E. blood vessels become narrow and obstruct the flow of blood to the heart

F. raw and inflamed skin rash, abdominal pain, diarrhea, dementia, and paralysis

G. bleeding gums, loss of teeth, internal bleeding, and anemia

H. porous, brittle bones

I. discolored skin, body sores, a bulging abdomen, and listlessness

J. abnormally large red blood cells and neurological disturbances, such as depression and drowsiness

K. swelling caused by build up of fluids

L. crooked legs, misshapen breast bone

M. cavities in the teeth

Nutrition Maze

Activity C   Name_____

Chapter 2   Date _____ Period _____

Read the definitions and write the corresponding terms in the blanks. Then find the terms in the word maze and circle them. (Terms are located forward, backward, horizontally, vertically, and diagonally in the maze.)

```
G A T R A C E Y O S A S E D I R A H C C A S O N O M
A D A Q R A E H T A E Z P I C K R C S L I F E O U D
S I G X E S P N T T J L U S J B M B E S R S I N C N
T A C C D N E G T U V O U A Q O E N E T O R A C T O
R A H A E I F I F I F N C O M P L E T E N T D B E I
I B W G R C H E R L B O N M I N C O M P L E T E T
C O F T J B L H W I X R I N D P Q C R U I X I W C A
J K U L D P O X G S M Z M A M I N O A C I D S E N N
U N U V N E T H E I N O I T I R T U N L A M V V M E
I Q C J K J T M Y Y L V T S D I P I L H O U A O E G
C E A H U A I K R D U M Q E P A W L W K C R G F T O
E I L C O D N D I S R J T A U S B P R O T E I N A R
S R C K L L G H C T X A U Y L R N Y O J O W B E B D
B M I I M P E L N W R K T K B Q V I X N Z S I V O Y
Q H U A U Q O S B U R J P E U G F S M Y L C X B L H
E N M P O E T Q T Y S F Z K S A H T V A I U U G I E
Z S O P E G V A C E E O W K T D E C R U T J Z Y S B
Y H C R A T S E Q Y R R T E W A T E R H Z I S D M R
P G Y Y F N F T N S I O E A L T N Y W D C J V Y E A
O L A A U D S N Z H N R L V L I M I W G P X Z X E F
S A T U R A T E D M E M Z U M U X L B L E E D I N G
```

1. _____ is the most abundant mineral found in the body.

2. _____ is the mineral that combines with a protein to form hemoglobin.

3. _____ are the simplest carbohydrates.

4. ___ _____ contain hydrochloric acid and several enzymes that break down food in the stomach.

5. _____ describes the chemical processes nutrients undergo once they have been absorbed into the body.

1. _____

2. _____

3. _____

4. _____

5. _____

Name _____

6. _____ is poor nutrition over an extended period of time.

6. _____

7. _____ is the unit of measurement used in nutrition to measure food energy.

7. _____

8. _____ are inorganic substances that account for approximately four percent of your body weight.

8. _____

9. _____ elements are those found in very small amounts in the body.

9. _____

10. _____-soluble vitamins must be supplied on a daily basis since they are not stored in the body.

10. _____

11. _____-soluble vitamins can be stored in the body.

11. _____

12. _____ is needed by the body for growth, maintenance, and repair of body tissues and for the formation of antibodies.

12. _____

13. _____ _____ are chemical compounds that are the building blocks of proteins.

13. _____

14. _____ proteins contain all eight essential amino acids, will support growth and normal maintenance of body tissues, and are found in foods of animal origin.

14. _____

15. _____ proteins lack one or more essential amino acids, will neither support growth nor provide for normal maintenance of body tissues, and are found in most plant foods.

15. _____

16. _____ fats are usually solid at room temperature.

16. _____

17. _____ fats are usually liquid at room temperature.

17. _____

18. _____ is a fatlike substance that has been linked with heart disease.

18. _____

19. _____ are the body's chief source of energy.

19. _____

20. _____ are chemical substances in foods that nourish the body, regulate bodily processes, and build cells and tissues.

20. _____

21. _____ are a group of compounds that include both fats and oils.

21. _____

22. _____ are complex organic substances needed in small amounts for normal growth, maintenance, and reproduction.

22. _____

23. _____ helps convert a substance found in the skin to vitamin D.

23. _____

24. _____ of blood, by helping the liver to make prothrombin, is an important function of vitamin K.

24. _____

25. _____ gums, bruising, loss of teeth, weight loss, soreness in joints, and scurvy can be caused by a deficiency of vitamin C.

25. _____

26. _____, found in dark green and yellow fruits and vegetables, can be converted into vitamin A by the body.

26. _____

27. _____ is the most abundant carbohydrate in the body.

27. _____

28. _____ is a process by which hydrogen is chemically added to an unsaturated fat.

28. _____

How the Body Uses Food

Activity D   Name _____

Chapter 2   Date _____ Period _____

Answer the following questions related to energy needs and the processes of digestion, absorption, and metabolism.

1. What is peristalsis? _____

   _____

2. What role do enzymes play in the process of digestion? _____

   _____

3. Place numbers in the blanks to indicate the order in which the following nutrients leave the stomach during digestion.

   _____ proteins   _____ fats   _____ carbohydrates

4. Using Appendix B (Nutritive Values of Foods) on pages 617 to 634 of the text, record the protein, fat, and carbohydrate content of the foods below.

	Protein (Grams)	Fat (Grams)	Carbohydrate (Grams)
1-inch cube Cheddar cheese	_____	_____	_____
apple	_____	_____	_____
roasted chicken drumstick	_____	_____	_____

5. If you were to choose one of the above foods for a snack, which one would satisfy your hunger the longest? Explain your answer. _____

   _____

   _____

6. Where does most absorption take place? _____

7. What are villi and what role do they play in the process of absorption? _____

   _____

8. Where do metabolic reactions take place? _____

9. Give an example of how each of the following nutrients could be used as a result of metabolic reactions.

   Carbohydrates: _____

   Fats: _____

   Proteins: _____

10. In each of the following pairs, place a check beside the description of the person who is likely to have the higher basal metabolic rate.

   A. _____ 5'10" tall person   _____ 6'1" tall person

   B. _____ male   _____ female

   C. _____ 15-year-old   _____ 30-year-old

   D. _____ a person with a body temperature   _____ a person with a body temperature
            of 98.6°F   of 101.2°F

Making Healthy Food Choices

What's Behind the Dietary Guidelines?

Activity A

Chapter 3

Name _____

Date _____ Period _____

The seven Dietary Guidelines for Americans are listed below. In the space provided, explain why each guideline was established.

1. Eat a variety of foods.

   _____

   _____

   _____

2. Balance the food you eat with physical activity—maintain or improve your weight.

   _____

   _____

   _____

3. Choose a diet with plenty of grain products, vegetables, and fruits.

   _____

   _____

   _____

4. Choose a diet low in fat, saturated fat, and cholesterol.

   _____

   _____

   _____

5. Choose a diet moderate in sugars.

   _____

   _____

   _____

6. Choose a diet moderate in salt and sodium.

   _____

   _____

   _____

7. If you drink alcoholic beverages, do so in moderation.

   _____

   _____

   _____

Do You Follow the Pyramid?

Activity B   Name _____

Chapter 3   Date _____ Period _____

Complete the chart below to see how your diet compares with the Food Guide Pyramid. Follow these steps:

1. List all the foods and beverages you consumed for one day. Be sure to include foods consumed as snacks as well as meals.
2. Note the amount of each food you eat.
3. Indicate the number of servings provided by each food under the correct food group heading. (You may wish to refer to page 57 in the text for information about typical serving sizes.) Since there are no typical serving sizes for fats, oils, and sweets, simply place a check (✓) in that column beside appropriate foods.
4. Use Appendix B (Nutritive Values of Foods) on pages 617 to 634 of the text to list the calorie and fat content of the foods and beverages you listed.
5. Add the total number of servings for each group, the total number of calories, and the total grams of fat.
6. Use the chart to complete the analysis that follows.

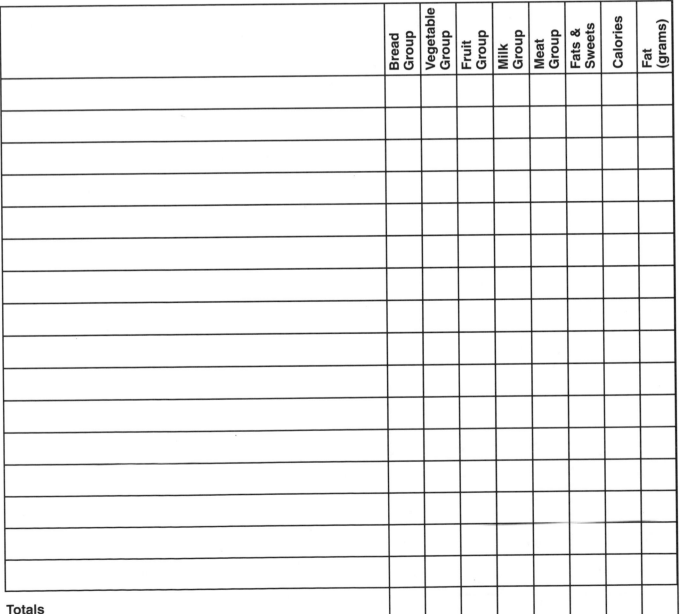

	Bread Group	Vegetable Group	Fruit Group	Milk Group	Meat Group	Fats & Sweets	Calories	Fat (grams)
Totals								

(Continued)

Name _____

From Chart 3-4 on page 58 of the text, indicate the daily number of calories, food group servings, and fat grams that would be appropriate for you. Then record the totals you consumed from the chart on the previous page.

	Calories	Bread Group	Vegetable Group	Fruit Group	Milk Group	Meat Group	Total Fat (grams)
Recommended	____	____	____	____	____	____	____
Consumed	____	____	____	____	____	____	____

1. Did you consume more or less than the recommended number of calories? _____

   _____

   What could result from following an eating pattern like this over a period of time? _____

   _____

2. Did you consume more or less than the recommended number of grams of fat? _____

   _____

   What could result from following an eating pattern like this over a period of time? _____

   _____

3. For what food groups did you consume more than the recommended number of servings? _____

   _____

   What could result from following an eating pattern like this over a period of time? _____

   _____

   What foods could you delete from your diet that would allow you to meet the recommended number of servings? _____

   _____

4. For what food groups did you consume less than the recommended number of servings? _____

   _____

   What could result from following an eating pattern like this over a period of time? _____

   _____

   What foods could you add to your diet that would allow you to meet the recommended number of servings? _____

   _____

Choosing Wisely When Shopping

Activity C   Name_____

Chapter 3   Date _____ Period _____

Read the following statements about purchasing food. Circle T if the statement is true, and circle F if the statement is false.

T   F   1. In most cases, processing decreases the nutritional value of foods.

T   F   2. Fresh foods are often more economical than processed foods.

T   F   3. Canned vegetables are lower in sodium than fresh vegetables.

T   F   4. Fruit juices are higher in fiber than fresh fruits.

T   F   5. Round steak and pork tenderloin are lean cuts of meat.

T   F   6. Dark meat pieces of chicken and turkey are lower in fat than light meat pieces.

T   F   7. Most varieties of fresh fish and shellfish are low in fat.

T   F   8. Nuts and seeds are lowfat meat alternates.

T   F   9. Nutritional labeling can help you compare similar products and different brands of the same product.

T   F   10. Whole grain bread and cereal products are high in fiber.

T   F   11. English muffins are a good source of complex carbohydrates, but they are also high in fat.

T   F   12. Although many breakfast cereals are good sources of fiber, some are high in added sugar and sodium.

T   F   13. Instant hot cereals tend to be much lower in sodium than regular and quick-cooking products.

T   F   14. Fruits canned in juice or water are lower in sugar than those canned in syrup.

T   F   15. Some fruit drinks and fruit punches may contain very little fruit juice.

T   F   16. Beans, peas, and lentils are lowfat, high-fiber meat alternates.

T   F   17. Most processed meats, like luncheon meats and hot dogs, are low in fat but high in sodium.

T   F   18. Fish canned in water is lower in fat than fish canned in oil.

T   F   19. Frozen yogurt is lower in fat than ice cream.

T   F   20. Many soups, sauce mixes, and packaged entrees are high in sodium.

T   F   21. An oatmeal raisin cookie is likely to be a more nutritious choice than a chocolate sandwich cookie with cream filling.

T   F   22. A margarine that lists a solid vegetable shortening as the first ingredient is a good choice for a product low in saturated fats.

Preparing Healthful Food

Activity D   Name _____

Chapter 3   Date _____ Period _____

Answer the following questions about preparing foods based on the Dietary Guidelines for Americans.

1. What is the advantage of preparing foods from scratch?

   _____

   _____

2. How should meat and poultry be prepared before cooking?

   _____

   _____

3. How large is a 3-ounce (84 g) portion of meat, poultry, or fish?

   _____

   _____

4. What might you serve for an entree if you were planning to serve chocolate caramel cheesecake for dessert?

   _____

   _____

5. How can you reduce the fat when preparing packaged pasta, rice, stuffing, and sauce mixes?

   _____

   _____

6. What can you do to reduce the fat added by such toppings as salad dressings, mayonnaise, sour cream, and cream cheese?

   _____

   _____

7. How can you limit your sodium and fat intake when preparing vegetables?

   _____

   _____

8. What modifications should be made to a recipe calling for cheese or condensed soup?

   _____

   _____

9. What other modifications might you make to a cake recipe in which you wanted to reduce the sugar?

   _____

   _____

10. How can you prepare egg dishes, such as omelets and scrambled eggs, while still limiting your cholesterol intake?

   _____

   _____

Dining Habits Survey

Activity E

Chapter 3

Name _____

Date _____ Period _____

Survey five teens about their habits and preferences when dining out. Record their answers in the chart provided. Then use your survey findings to make a general recommendation for teens regarding their food choices when eating out.

1. What is your sex?   A. male   B. female
2. How often do you eat away from home?   A. less than once a week   B. once a week   C. two to three times a week   D. four to five times a week   E. once a day   F. more than once a day
3. Where do you most often get the food you eat away from home?   A. fast-food restaurants   B. school cafeteria   C. sit-down restaurants   D. pizza parlors and/or sandwich shops   E. snack bars and concession stands   F. vending machines   G. convenience or grocery stores   H. friends' homes
4. What types of foods do you most often choose when you eat away from home?   A. hamburgers and other sandwiches   B. pizza   C. chips and other salty snacks   D. fried foods   E. candy, ice cream, desserts, or other sweets   F. soft drinks and shakes
5. What impact does nutritional value have on your food choices when eating out?   A. a great deal of impact   B. some impact   C. little impact   D. no impact
6. Who do you usually eat with when you eat away from home?   A. family members   B. friends   C. dating partner   D. coworkers   E. I usually eat alone.
7. Why do you usually eat away from home?   A. convenience   B. entertainment   C. variety   D. to be with friends   E. to avoid cooking   F. habit
8. What factor has the greatest influence on the foods you choose?   A. cost   B. personal likes and dislikes   C. nutrition   D. choices of people eating with me

Survey Responses

Question	Person 1	Person 2	Person 3	Person 4	Person 5
1.					
2.					
3.					
4.					
5.					
6.					
7.					
8.					

What conclusions can you draw from your survey findings? _____

_____

_____

What recommendation would you make to teens about their food choices when eating out based on these conclusions? _____

_____

_____

Nutrition Through the Life Cycle

Baby Food

Activity A

Chapter 4

Name _____

Date _____ Period _____

Interview the mother of an infant. Record her responses to the questions below.

1. How much weight did you gain during your pregnancy? _____

2. Was your weight gain within your obstetrician's recommendations? _____

3. What changes did you make in your diet when you were pregnant? _____
_____

4. What, if any, dietary supplements did your obstetrician prescribe during your pregnancy? _____
_____

5. How old is your baby? _____

6. How much did your child weigh at birth? _____

   How much does your child weigh now? _____

   What is the weight increase or decrease? _____

7. How long was your child at birth? _____

   How long is your child now? _____

   What is the length increase? _____

8. Is your baby breast-fed or formula-fed? _____

9. How many times a day do you feed your baby? _____

10. What do you feed your baby besides milk? _____
_____

11. How much milk and solid food does your baby consume each day? _____
_____

12. What, if any, dietary supplements has your pediatrician recommended for your baby? _____
_____

13. When did you, or at what age do you plan to, introduce solid foods into your baby's diet? _____
_____

14. What solid foods did or will you introduce first? _____
_____

15. What procedure has your pediatrician recommended for introducing new foods to your baby?
_____
_____

Making a Weight Management Plan

Activity B   Name_____

Chapter 4   Date _____ Period _____

Analyze the menus below and consider how you would alter them to help an adult lose weight. Then complete this activity following the steps below.

Breakfast	Calories	Fat (g)
1. Orange juice from concentrate, ¾ cup (175 mL)	83	0
2. Granola, 1 ounce (28 g)	125	5
3. Whole milk, ½ cup (125 mL)	75	8
4. Coffee, with sugar	15	0
Lunch		
5. Oil pack tuna, 3 ounces (84 g)	165	7
6. White bread, 2 slices (18 per loaf)	130	2
7. Tossed salad greens, 1 cup (250 mL)	5	0
8. Thousand Island dressing, 1 tablespoon (15 mL)	60	6
9. Whole milk, 1 cup (250 mL)	150	8
10. Chocolate chip cookies, 4 medium	180	9
Dinner		
11. Broiled steak, 3 ounces (84 g)	240	15
12. Baked potato, 1 medium with skin	220	0
13. Sour cream, 1 tablespoon (15 mL)	25	3
14. Steamed broccoli, ½ cup (125 mL)	23	0
15. Cheese sauce, 2 tablespoons (30 mL)	38	2
16. Dinner roll, 1 small	85	2
17. Butter, 1 teaspoon (5 mL)	35	4
18. Vanilla ice cream, 1 cup (250 mL)	270	14
19. Iced tea, with sugar	30	0
Snack		
20. Chocolate bar with almonds, 2 ounces (60 g)	300	20
	2254	105

1. In the first, second, third, and fourth columns of the chart on the next page, list the item number, name, calorie value, and fat value of each food you would eliminate or replace in the menus above.
2. In the fifth column, list foods you would substitute opposite those you are replacing. Leave this column blank opposite foods you are eliminating. (When selecting substitutes, remember to choose foods of similar or greater nutritive value than those you are replacing. Be sure to include the minimum recommended number of servings from each food group in your adapted menus.)
3. Use Appendix B (Nutritive Values of Foods) on pages 617 to 634 of the text to determine the calorie and fat values of the foods you are substituting. List those values in the last two columns.
4. Compute the total calorie and fat savings.
5. Answer the questions below the chart.

(Continued)

Name _____

Item Number	Foods Being Replaced or Eliminated	Calorie Values	Fat Values	Substitute Foods	Calorie Values	Fat Values

Total calories of replaced or eliminated foods   _____

Total calories of substitute foods   – _____

Total calorie savings   _____

Total grams of fat in replaced or eliminated foods   _____

Total grams of fat in substitute foods   – _____

Total grams of fat saved   _____

1. Identify five hazards of being obese. _____
   _____
   _____
   _____

2. Identify two causes of overweight. _____
   _____
   _____

3. Give two tips for successful weight loss. _____
   _____
   _____

4. What five factors affect your daily calorie need?_____
   _____
   _____

5. Explain the basics of planning a good weight management plan. ____
   _____
   _____

Diets in the Life Cycle

Activity C   Name _____

Chapter 4   Date _____ Period _____

Answer the questions related to changing dietary needs throughout the life cycle based on the menus below.

Breakfast

¾ cup (175 mL) orange juice   1 cup (250 mL) coffee
2 slices French toast with
   1 tablespoon (15 mL) syrup

Lunch

1 cup (250 mL) chili made with   2 slices whole wheat bread
   ground beef and kidney beans   ½ cup canned peaches
½ cup (125 mL) corn   1 cup (250 mL) lowfat milk

Dinner

3 ounces (84 g) ham   1 square cornbread with 1 teaspoon
½ cup (125 mL) carrots   (5 mL) margarine
   small salad with 1 tablespoon   1 slice cheesecake
   (15 mL) French dressing   1 cup (250 mL) lowfat milk

1. How might a pregnant woman modify these menus to meet her special nutritional needs?

   _____

   _____

2. What foods could you substitute in this lunch menu that would appeal more to a preschooler? Explain your answer. _____

   _____

   _____

3. What foods could you substitute in this breakfast menu that would appeal to a school-age child who does not like traditional breakfast foods? _____

   _____

   _____

4. What kinds of snack foods could you add to these menus to meet the increased nutritional needs of a teenager? (Keep in mind the recommended number of servings teens should have from each food group.)

   _____

   _____

5. What foods could you substitute in these menus to meet the calcium needs of an older adult who does not like to drink milk?_____

   _____

6. What foods could you substitute in these menus to meet the protein needs of a lacto-ovo vegetarian?

   _____

   _____

Nutrition Advice

Activity D   Name _____

Chapter 4   Date _____ Period _____

Pretend you write a column called, "The Diet Counselor," for a local newspaper. Use chapter information to answer the following letters from your readers about their nutrition concerns.

Dear Diet Counselor,
*   Since learning last week that my wife is preg-*
nant, I've been cooking up a storm. I've been
making big breakfasts, big lunches, big dinners,
and big snacks. Despite my efforts, she's eating
no more now than she did before getting preg-
nant. I'm afraid she's not getting enough nutrients
for the baby. Please advise.
*   Expectant Father*

1. Dear Dad,

_____

_____

_____

_____

_____

_____

_____

_____

                    D.C.

Dear Diet Counselor,
*   My three-year-old son is a finicky eater. At*
some meals, he barely eats at all. Should I be
concerned?
*   Muddled Mom*

2. Dear Muddled,

_____

_____

_____

_____

_____

_____

_____

_____

                    D.C.

Dear Diet Counselor,
*   After my parents leave for work, I'm in charge*
of getting my nine-year-old brother off to school.
He doesn't really like cereal and toast, so most
mornings he just skips breakfast. Is this okay?
*   Big Brother*

3. Dear Brother,

_____

_____

_____

_____

_____

_____

_____

_____

                    D.C.

Dear Diet Counselor,
*   One of my friends told me he is a "lacto-ovo"*
vegetarian. What does this mean?
*   A Meat Lover*

4. Dear Meat Lover,

_____

_____

_____

_____

_____

_____

_____

_____

                    D.C.   *(Continued)*

Name _____

Dear Diet Counselor,

My grandmother has brittle bones. Someone told me this is caused by a poor diet. Is there something my grandmother could eat to make her bones stronger? Will I suffer from brittle bones when I am her age?

A Concerned
Granddaughter

5. Dear Concerned,

_____
_____
_____
_____
_____
_____
_____
_____

D.C.

Dear Diet Counselor,

I'm on the school football team. I eat a high protein diet to help build my strength and keep up my energy. Should I also be using nutrient supplements?

Future Pro Player

7. Dear Pro,

_____
_____
_____
_____
_____
_____
_____
_____

D.C.

Dear Diet Counselor,

My job, family, and community activities keep me pretty busy. I find myself relying on fast-food restaurants for many of my meals. As a result, I've started to put on a little unwanted weight. What can I do to improve my diet?

Middle-Aged Bulge

6. Dear Bulge,

_____
_____
_____
_____
_____
_____
_____

D.C.

Dear Diet Counselor,

I'm worried about my older sister. She eats like a pig, and then she makes herself throw up. She says she's got the best of both worlds—she can eat all she wants and not gain an ounce. Is what she's doing healthy?

Little Sis

8. Dear Sis,

_____
_____
_____
_____
_____
_____
_____
_____

D.C.

Safeguarding the Family's Health

Kitchen Sanitation

Activity A

Chapter 5

Name _____

Date _____ Period _____

Read the following story. In the space provided at the bottom of the page, list 10 guidelines of personal and kitchen cleanliness that Gina failed to follow.

A Not-so-Safe Supper

Gina came into the house and set the tomatoes she had just picked on the kitchen counter. She'd been working in the garden all afternoon and had lost track of time. Now Gina was getting a late start preparing dinner. She decided to get the meatloaf into the oven before she went upstairs to shower and change.

Gina needed a large bowl in which to mix her ingredients. As she bent over to get one out of the cabinet, her long hair tumbled over her shoulders. Gina quickly brushed her hair aside with her hands and went about her work.

Gina got the ground beef out of the refrigerator, unwrapped it, and put it in the bowl. Then she got an onion out of a sack under the kitchen sink. As Gina started chopping the onion, some of the juice got into a cut on her finger and made her wince in pain.

Gina mixed the chopped onion and other ingredients with the ground beef in the bowl. Then she turned the mixture out onto a cutting board and shaped it into a loaf with her hands. Gina put the meatloaf in a baking pan and put it in the oven.

Gina wiped her hands on a dish towel. Then she got the lettuce out of the refrigerator to make a salad.

Gina tore the lettuce into a bowl. She cut one of the tomatoes from the garden on the cutting board she'd used for the meatloaf. Gina arranged the tomato wedges on top of the lettuce and put the salad in the refrigerator.

Just then, Gina's dog came into the kitchen. "I guess it's time for your dinner, too," Gina said. She opened a can of dog food and emptied it into his dish beside the refrigerator.

Gina found a can of spaghetti sauce on the pantry shelf that she thought would taste good on the meatloaf. She blew the dust off the top of the can and opened it.

As Gina was pouring the sauce in a pan to heat, she spilled some of it on the counter. She decided to leave the spill, along with the dirty dishes, to clean up later. With only 30 minutes until the meatloaf would be done, Gina went upstairs to take a shower.

1. _____
2. _____
3. _____
4. _____
5. _____
6. _____
7. _____
8. _____
9. _____
10. _____

Sanitation in Food Preparation and Storage

Activity B   Name _____

Chapter 5   Date _____ Period _____

1. Using a contrasting color, mark the bacterial growth danger zone.

Temperatures	**Deg. F**
Canning	
───────────────────────────────	212 ─
Heating and warming	
───────────────────────────────	126 ─
Room	
───────────────────────────────	60 ─
Refrigerator	
───────────────────────────────	32 ─
Freezer	

2. Why are temperatures in this zone called the *danger zone*?

_____

_____

3. What is the maximum amount of time perishable foods can safely be held in the danger zone?

_____

_____

4. What guidelines should be followed when serving foods to prevent bacteria from multiplying rapidly?

_____

_____

5. How should foods be packaged for the freezer? _____

_____

_____

6. How should low-acid, home-canned foods be prepared? _____

_____

_____

7. How should leftovers be prepared? _____

_____

_____

8. What guidelines should be followed when stuffing raw poultry, meat, or fish? _____

_____

_____

Safety Is No Accident

Activity C   Name _____

Chapter 5   Date _____ Period _____

Evaluate your knowledge of kitchen safety as you play the game below. Use buttons, circles of paper, or coins for markers and flip a coin to move around the board. If the coin is flipped "heads," move the marker two spaces. If the coin is flipped "tails," move the marker one space. The player who finishes first is the winner.

1. START

2. You remembered to put on rubber gloves before picking up broken glass. Move ahead 1 space.

3. Cuts

4. You disconnect appliances by pulling on the cord. Move back 1 space.

8. Burns & Fires

7. You sat your toaster near a puddle of water on the counter. Go back to start.

6.

5. You have a fire extinguisher in your kitchen. Take another turn.

9. You remember to turn pan handles inward on the range to avoid accidental tipping. Move ahead 2 spaces.

18. Your kitchen knives are dull. Miss a turn while you sharpen them.

17.

16. Your kitchen floor is free from throw rugs and other objects. Move ahead 1 space.

10. You left cabinet doors hanging open. Miss a turn to give yourself a chance to close them.

19.

20. FINISH **Congratulations!** You've shown that you can work safely in the kitchen.

15. You tell a friend a joke just as he takes a bite of food, causing him to start choking. Move back to space 10.

11.

12. You stood on a chair to reach a high shelf. Move back 1 space.

13. You have a poison chart posted in your medicine cabinet. Take another turn.

14. Falls

Handling Emergencies

Activity D

Chapter 5

Name _____

Date _____ Period _____

Indicate the most appropriate response to each of the following emergency situations.

1. You get a minor cut on your knuckle while grating cheese. What do you do? _____

_____

_____

2. You burn the back of your hand on an oven rack. What do you do? _____

_____

_____

3. Your mother falls off of a step stool and you think her ankle may be broken. What do you do?

_____

_____

_____

4. A child in your care has just swallowed some type of cleaning fluid in an unlabeled bottle. What do you do?

_____

_____

_____

5. You find your sister lying on the kitchen floor. A portable mixer, still plugged in, is in the sink and the water is running. You suspect your sister has received an electric shock. What do you do?

_____

_____

_____

6. You are having dinner with a friend when she suddenly puts her hand to her throat. She cannot speak and her face is beginning to turn blue. What do you do? _____

_____

_____

7. You gash your wrist with a cleaver. Blood is spurting out of the deep wound. What do you do?

_____

_____

_____

8. Your grandmother serves chicken for dinner. Later, she complains of a severe headache, abdominal pain, and vomiting. You suspect she is suffering from salmonellosis. What do you do?

_____

_____

Career Opportunities

Chapter 6

Career Self-Analysis

Activity A

Name _____

Chapter 6

Date _____ Period _____

Complete the chart below by listing your likes, dislikes, interests, and abilities in the appropriate columns. Then answer the questions that follow.

Likes	Dislikes	Interests	Abilities

1. Do you like to work with people? _____

2. Are you artistic? _____

3. Do you like to write? _____

4. Do you consider yourself to be a leader? _____

5. Do you like to travel? _____

6. What do you plan to do after graduating from high school? _____
   _____

7. What career do you think you might be interested in pursuing? _____
   _____

8. How does this career correspond with the likes, dislikes, interests, and abilities you listed in the chart above? _____
   _____
   _____

9. From whom can you obtain information about your career interests? List three. _____
   _____
   _____

10. What types of work experiences (part-time jobs, clubs, activities, etc.) could you get involved in now that relate to your career interest? _____
    _____
    _____

Career Maze

Activity B   Name _____

Chapter 6   Date _____ Period _____

Complete the statements by writing terms related to careers in the blanks. Then find the terms in the word maze and circle them. (Terms are located forward, backward, horizontally, vertically, and diagonally in the maze.)

```
K  U  M  E  T  S  I  N  O  I  T  I  R  T  U  N  C  N  W  A
M  T  L  C  A  L  B  R  S  A  N  I  T  A  T  I  O  N  N  U
A  D  M  I  N  I  S  T  R  A  T  I  O  N  G  I  M  H  A  E
A  N  K  V  C  I  O  S  Q  O  X  F  E  U  T  K  M  B  L  L
F  S  T  R  E  D  D  A  L  R  E  E  R  A  C  B  U  J  J  R
F  J  I  E  O  N  P  L  E  E  I  V  R  H  U  J  N  U  T  T
A  O  D  S  R  S  R  I  A  F  F  A  F  S  S  I  I  B  O  E
Y  E  R  D  L  N  D  N  D  M  P  T  I  I  T  V  C  S  M  C
M  H  U  O  N  A  B  A  E  E  L  N  S  G  O  C  A  H  V  M
A  A  E  O  B  I  Q  E  R  E  E  I  D  G  M  A  T  N  E  B
H  N  N  F  Z  T  F  P  E  S  K  Z  N  K  E  W  I  U  C  S
A  D  E  A  O  I  W  J  S  Y  M  I  B  T  R  M  O  E  N  E
I  L  R  P  G  T  E  D  A  X  H  N  Y  L  E  T  N  I  E  R
M  I  P  P  Q  E  R  R  H  C  R  A  E  S  E  R  S  E  R  A
Z  N  E  R  C  I  M  S  A  Y  T  Z  O  X  R  N  V  F  E  C
G  G  R  B  X  D  V  E  U  C  E  U  O  V  P  E  D  I  F  L
A  Y  T  G  E  X  T  E  N  S  I  O  N  X  C  S  S  G  E  H
V  H  N  F  G  N  I  R  E  T  A  C  O  D  I  V  Q  E  R  W
A  R  E  W  D  I  D  E  P  Z  N  W  G  Q  N  R  E  A  R  N
```

1. A series of related jobs that form a career is a _____.

2. A person who commands authority and takes a principal role in a group is a _____.

3. Food preparation, customer service, sanitation, and management are the four areas of careers in the _____ _____ industry.

4. Making soup, helping with breakfast orders, and assisting a grill cook are examples of tasks someone might perform in the food _____ area of food service.

5. The _____ service area of food service involves working with the people a food establishment serves.

6. The _____ area of food service involves cleaning and maintenance.

1. _____

2. _____

3. _____

4. _____

5. _____

6. _____

(Continued)

Name _____

7. Positions in the _____ area of food service include owner, manager, and executive chef.

7. _____

8. A business that combines all four areas of food service is _____.

8. _____

9. Careers in the food _____ industry involve harvesting, processing, and selling food products.

9. _____

10. Professionals who work in the field of _____ lead food classes for people at all educational levels.

10. _____

11. _____ agents work with adults and with young people involved in 4-H programs.

11. _____

12. _____ are members of the health care team who have special knowledge and training in food and nutrition, the health sciences, and institution management.

12. _____

13. Dietitians who work in the area of nutritional _____ work for hospitals, clinics, and nursing homes.

13. _____

14. Dietitians who work in the area of _____ plan meals, supervise and train personnel, and oversee the purchase of food and equipment.

14. _____

15. A registered dietitian or a family and consumer science professional with a degree in foods and nutrition is a _____.

15. _____

16. Food professionals in _____ usually work with the mass media.

16. _____

17. Food professionals in _____ are hired by private companies, associations, and utility companies.

17. _____

18. A person with a career in consumer _____ answers consumer questions and investigates complaints.

18. _____

19. Nutrition studies, equipment development, and product testing are some of the tasks in which a food professional in _____ might be involved.

19. _____

20. Someone other than a friend or relative that an employer can call to ask about a job applicant's capabilities as a worker is a _____.

20. _____

21. An opportunity for an employer and a job applicant to discuss the applicant's qualifications is a(n) _____.

21. _____

22. Someone who sets up and runs his or her own business is a(n) _____.

22. _____

Careers in Foods

Activity C   Name _____

Chapter 6   Date _____ Period _____

Answer the following questions in the space provided.

1. Define *food service industry.*

   _____

   _____

2. List the four areas of food service and give an example of a job in each area.

Area	Career
_____	_____
_____	_____
_____	_____
_____	_____

3. Investigate and describe the job requirements for one of the food service positions you listed above.

   _____

   _____

4. Define *food handling industry.*

   _____

   _____

5. List five jobs in the food handling industry.

   _____

   _____

6. Investigate and describe the job requirements for one of the food handling positions you listed above.

   _____

   _____

7. Briefly describe the seven types of food-related careers in education and business.

   _____

   _____

   _____

   _____

   _____

8. Investigate and describe the job requirements of one of the types of food-related careers in education and business.

   _____

   _____

Application Information

Activity D

Chapter 6

Name _____

Date _____ Period _____

Consider how you would fill out a job application form by completing the personal fact sheet below. Then answer the questions that follow.

Personal Fact Sheet

Social Security number _____-_____-_____

Name _____
       Last   First   Middle initial

Address _____
           Street   City   State   Zip code

Telephone ___(____)_____
            Area Code

Education

	Name & Location	Years Completed	Subjects Studied	Grade Average
Elementary School				
Junior High School				
High School				

Additional coursework _____

Work Experience

Employer_____Supervisor _____

Address _____
            Street   City   State   Zip code

Telephone ___(____)_____Employed from_____to _____
            Area Code

Job title _____Salary range _____to _____

Duties_____

Employer_____Supervisor _____

Address _____
            Street   City   State   Zip code

Telephone ___(____)_____Employed from_____to _____
            Area Code

Job title _____Salary range _____to _____

Duties_____

References

Name _____Relationship _____

Address _____
            Street   City   State   Zip code

Telephone ___(____)_____Years acquainted_____
            Area Code

Name _____Relationship _____

Address _____
            Street   City   State   Zip code

Telephone ___(____)_____Years acquainted_____
            Area Code

---

1. For what types of positions would you be interested in applying? _____

   _____

2. What hobbies or special skills do you have that might relate to these types of jobs? _____

   _____

3. What honors and awards have you received that might impress an employer in an interview? _____

   _____

4. How much money would you expect to earn when you start a part-time job? _____

You're the Boss

Activity E   Name _____

Chapter 6   Date _____ Period _____

Explore your interest in becoming an entrepreneur by completing this worksheet to plan a food-related business.

1. What would you name your business? _____

2. What type of business would this be? _____

3. What types of food products or food-related services would you provide?_____
_____

4. Where would your business be located?_____

5. Why do you think this type of business would be successful in this area? _____
_____

6. Who would your customers be?_____

7. What other businesses would create competition for you? _____
_____

8. How would you advertise your business? _____
_____

9. What type of equipment and supplies would you need to purchase to operate this business? _____
_____

10. Would you need to hire employees to help you run this business? _____ If so, how
many? _____

11. How much money do you think it would take to get this business started? (Don't forget to consider such expenses as rent, utilities, office supplies and equipment, accounting and legal fees, shipping and advertising costs, salaries, and taxes.) _____
_____

12. What kind of education and work experience could help you prepare to open this business? _____
_____

After answering the above questions, would you have any interest in exploring entrepreneurship further?
Explain why or why not._____
_____
_____
_____
_____
_____

Kitchen and Dining Areas Chapter **7**

Kitchen Floor Plans

Activity A

Chapter 7

Name _____

Date _____ Period _____

Complete the following exercises related to kitchen floor plans.

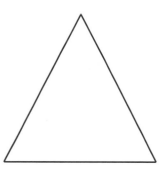

1. Label the three major work centers of the work triangle to the left.

2. What should the maximum total distance between the points of the work triangle be? _____

3. What additional work centers might be found in a kitchen? _____

_____

_____

4. Label each of the kitchen floor plans below and draw in the work triangle.

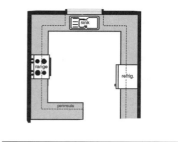
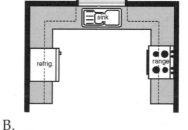
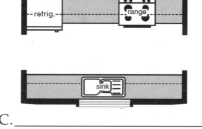

A. _____   B. _____   C. _____

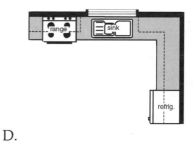
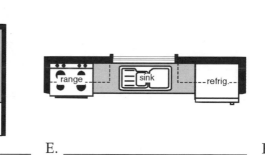
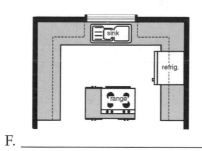

D. _____   E. _____   F. _____

5. Which plan is considered the most desirable? _____

   Why? _____

6. Which plan can easily include an eating area or another built-in appliance? _____

7. In which kitchen may traffic interfere with the work triangle? _____

8. Which plan is most often found in apartments? _____

   Name a disadvantage of this plan. _____

9. In which plan does a counter stand alone in the center of the room? _____

10. Which plan can easily adapt to a variety of room arrangements? _____

Kitchen and Dining Area Design Crossword

Activity B

Chapter 7

Name _____

Date _____ Period _____

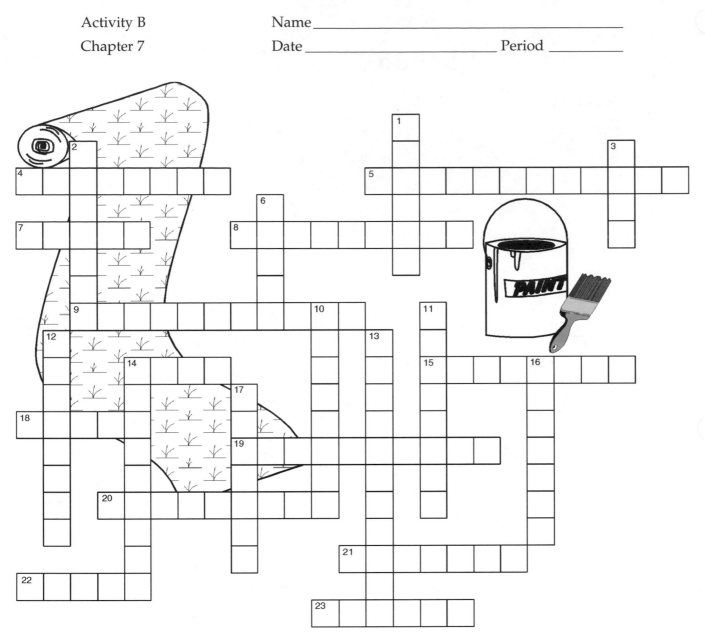

(Continued)

Name _____

Across

4. _____ _____ should be avoided on kitchen floors due to the danger of tripping.

5. Analyzing the room and establishing a budget should be done before beginning any _____.

7. _____ insets on cabinet doors allow china, crystal, and other stored items to be displayed.

8. Plastic _____ are popular for kitchen cabinets because they are colorful and easy to clean.

9. _____ provide work space in the kitchen and serving space in dining areas.

14. _____ flooring can be expensive, but its durability makes it economical.

15. If an appliance with a damaged wire is _____, the electric current will flow to the ground instead of through your body.

18. _____ wall coverings come in many patterns and can be wiped clean with a damp cloth.

19. _____ light most often comes from electrical fixtures.

20. _____ provides good walking comfort and reduces noise.

21. A small wire attached to a two-pronged adapter for grounded appliances is called a _____.

22. _____ coverings should provide walking comfort and be durable.

23. Cabinets made from wood _____ add warmth and natural beauty to a room.

Down

1. Vinyl _____ are popular on kitchen floors because they are durable and grease-resistant.

2. _____ tiles are a heatproof countertop material.

3. As a wall covering, _____ is used primarily in kitchens.

6. Semigloss _____ is best for kitchen walls because it can be washed easily.

10. _____ can be used to cover rough, unattractive walls in kitchen and dining areas.

11. Adequate _____ is needed to prevent kitchen accidents and to allow diners to see what they are eating.

12. _____ are needed in kitchen and dining areas to store such items as food, appliances, cleaning supplies, cooking utensils, dinnerware, and table decorations.

13. _____ is needed in a kitchen to remove steam, heat, and cooking odors.

14. _____ is a relatively inexpensive wall covering that is available in many colors and patterns.

16. _____ light comes from the sun.

17. Laminated _____ is often used for kitchen countertops because it is easy to clean, moisture-resistant, and durable.

Choosing Tableware

Activity C   Name _____

Chapter 7   Date _____ Period _____

Visit the tableware department in a department store. Select patterns of the types of tableware listed below that you like. Record the names of the patterns in the chart along with the names of the manu-facturers and pricing information. Then answer the questions that follow.

Dinnerware

Material	Pattern Name	Manufacturer	Sold (✓) OS	BTS*	Price per Place setting
China					
Stoneware					
Earthenware					
Pottery					
Glass ceramic					
Plastic					

Flatware

Sterling silver					
Silver plate					
Stainless steel					

Beverageware

Lead glass					
Lime glass					
Plastic					

*OS = open stock; BTS = by the set

1. Which of the above tableware items would you choose for formal dining?_____

   _____

   Why? _____

2. Which of the above tableware items would you choose for semiformal dining? _____

   _____

   Why? _____

3. Which of the above tableware items would you choose for casual dining? _____

   _____

   Why? _____

Setting the Table

Activity D   Name _____

Chapter 7   Date _____ Period _____

Using the rectangles below as place mats, draw an individual cover for each of the following menus. Each cover should include the correct placement of the dinnerware, flatware, glassware, and linens needed by one person. Label or draw the menu items for each cover as shown in the following example.

Steak
Baked Potato
Tossed Salad
Texas Toast
Strawberry Ice Cream
Iced Tea

Orange Juice
Oatmeal
Muffin
Milk

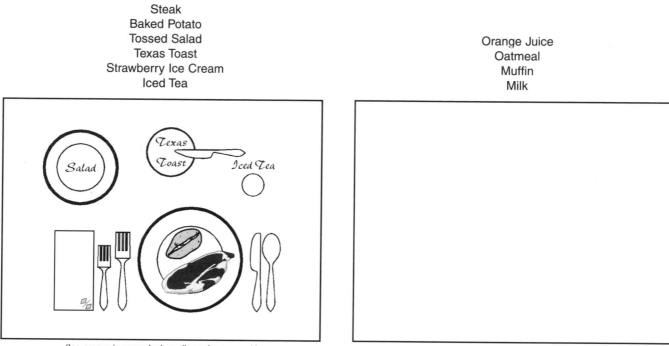

(Ice cream is served when dinner is removed.)

Tuna Sandwich
Celery and Carrot Sticks
Cookies
Milk

Barbecued Chicken
Mashed Potatoes Broccoli
Dinner Rolls
Apple Pie
Milk

Meal Service

Activity E   Name _____

Chapter 7   Date _____ Period _____

The six major styles of meal service are listed below. Read the following meal service descriptions. Then write the letter of the style of meal service to which it corresponds in the blank. (Some letters will be used more than once.)

A. American or family service
B. Russian or continental service
C. English service
D. compromise service
E. blue plate service
F. buffet service

_____   1. This style of service requires a great deal of passing plates at the table.

_____   2. A style of meal service in which guests serve themselves from a table that holds serving pieces and often holds tableware and napkins.

_____   3. Serving dishes are passed around the table, and family members and guests serve themselves.

_____   4. Serving dishes are never placed on the table.

_____   5. Food is placed in front of the host, and the plates are filled by the host and passed around the table until each guest has been served.

_____   6. This is the most formal style of meal service.

_____   7. This is the style of meal service used most often in the United States.

_____   8. This is a combination of Russian service and English service.

_____   9. Plates are filled in the kitchen, carried into the dining room, and served.

_____ 10. Guests are served filled plates of food by servants.

Read the following statements about waiting on the table. If the statement is true, circle *T*. If the statement is false, circle *F*.

T   F   11. The style of service helps determine the way in which the table is cleared and new courses are served.

T   F   12. The table is cleared in a clockwise direction.

T   F   13. The cohost is usually served first.

T   F   14. When serving, the server should stand at the guest's left side and place the plate with the left hand.

T   F   15. When clearing a course, the serving dishes should be removed first.

T   F   16. A small tray should be used to remove items that will not be needed for the next course.

T   F   17. Water is poured from the left side with the left hand.

T   F   18. When serving a new course, the first step is to place the needed dinnerware at each cover.

Choosing Kitchen Appliances

Major Appliance Shopper's Comparison

Activity A

Chapter 8

Name _____

Date _____ Period _____

Visit an appliance dealer and compare two different but comparable models of a major kitchen appliance. Fill in the information requested below and then complete the evaluation that follows.

Type of appliance _____

Appliance A

Brand _____

1. **Appliance Cost**
   - A. Appliance price $_____
   - B. Delivery cost   _____
   - C. Installation cost   _____
   - Total purchase cost $_____
2. **Service**
   - A. Will the dealer service the appliance in your home?

     _____
   - B. Warranty information—check all that apply.
     - _____ full
     - _____ limited
     - _____ entire appliance covered
     - _____ parts of appliance covered
     - _____ labor costs covered
     - How long is the warranty in effect?
   - C. Is a service contract available for this appliance?

     _____
     - What does it cover? _____
     _____
     _____
     _____
     - How long is it in effect? _____
     - How much does it cost?_____
3. **Operation**
   - What is the EnergyGuide rating (estimated yearly energy cost) of this appliance? _____

Appliance B

Brand _____

1. **Appliance Cost**
   - A. Appliance price $_____
   - B. Delivery cost   _____
   - C. Installation cost   _____
   - Total purchase cost $_____
2. **Service**
   - A. Will the dealer service the appliance in your home?

     _____
   - B. Warranty information—check all that apply.
     - _____ full
     - _____ limited
     - _____ entire appliance covered
     - _____ parts of appliance covered
     - _____ labor costs covered
     - How long is the warranty in effect?
   - C. Is a service contract available for this appliance?

     _____
     - What does it cover? _____
     _____
     _____
     _____
     - How long is it in effect? _____
     - How much does it cost?_____
3. **Operation**
   - What is the EnergyGuide rating (estimated yearly energy cost) of this appliance? _____

Based on the above purchase information, which of these two appliances would you buy? Explain your choice.

_____

_____

_____

_____

_____

Selecting Major Appliances

Activity B

Chapter 8

Name _____

Date _____ Period _____

Draw the Underwriters Laboratories (UL) seal and the blue star seal given by the American Gas Association (AGA). Label and explain the purpose of each.

Seal: _____   Seal: _____

Purpose: _____   Purpose: _____

_____   _____

_____   _____

Read the following statements about selecting appliances and equipment. If the statement is true, circle *T*. If the statement is false, circle *F*.

T   F   1. A limited warranty means that you can be charged for repairs, and you may have to return the appliance to the warrantor or take other steps to have it repaired.

T   F   2. While a full warranty is in effect, you can have an appliance repaired or replaced free of charge (at the warrantor's option) if it fails to operate properly.

T   F   3. A service contract is another name for a warranty.

T   F   4. EnergyGuide labels show an estimated yearly cost of running a major appliance.

T   F   5. The kind and size of the appliance needed may depend on the size of your family.

T   F   6. Space limitations are important points to consider when selecting an appliance.

T   F   7. When shopping for an appliance, visit several dealers to check both quality and price.

T   F   8. Installation and delivery costs may not be listed or included in the base price of an appliance.

T   F   9. Price is the major factor to consider when purchasing an appliance.

T   F   10. To cut costs, manufacturers are now offering fewer convenience features on major appliances than ever before.

T   F   11. Some consumers want compact appliance models that conserve space in smaller homes and apartments.

T   F   12. Electronics allow consumers to program appliances for specific tasks.

Microwave Survey

Activity C   Name _____

Chapter 8   Date _____ Period _____

Survey five people about their use of microwave ovens. Record their answers in the chart provided. Compile your results with those of your classmates. Write an article for your school paper reporting your findings.

1. What is your sex? A. male B. female

2. What is your age? A. under 12 B. 12 to 18 C. 18 to 30 D. Over 30

3. Are you the primary meal manager in your home? A. yes B. no

4. Do you have a microwave oven in your home? A. yes B. no (If no, answer only question 11.)

5. What style of microwave oven do you have? A. countertop B. over-the-range C. built-in D. under-the-cabinet

6. How often do you use your microwave oven? A. once a week B. two to three times a week C. four to five times a week D. daily

7. For what task do you most often use your microwave oven? A. defrosting frozen foods B. heating prepared foods C. cooking homemade foods D. reheating leftovers

8. What do you consider to be the greatest advantage of microwave cooking? A. faster cooking B. easy cleanup C. energy savings D. greater nutrition

9. Have you purchased any special cookware for use in your microwave oven? A. yes B. no

10. Do you feel you understand how a microwave oven works? A. yes B. no

11. Do you feel that microwave ovens are safe? A. yes B. no

12. Do you feel you use your microwave oven to its fullest advantage? A. yes B. no

Survey Responses

Question	Person 1	Person 2	Person 3	Person 4	Person 5
1.					
2.					
3.					
4.					
5.					
6.					
7.					
8.					
9.					
10.					
11.					
12.					

Portable Appliance Performance Comparison

Activity D   Name _____

Chapter 8   Date _____ Period _____

Choose two portable appliances that perform the same basic tasks. (Possible choices include standard mixer and hand mixer, blender and food processor, toaster and toaster-oven, and electric percolator and automatic drip coffeemaker.) Prepare the same simple food product with both appliances. Then complete the comparison below.

1. Food product prepared: _____

2. Preparation steps completed by the appliance: _____

     _____

3.

Appliance A _____	Appliance B _____
Convenience features	Convenience features
Safety features	Safety features
Advantages	Advantages
Disadvantages	Disadvantages

4. Which appliance do you feel did a better job of preparing the food product?_____

     Why? _____

5. For what types of food products might the other appliance be preferred?_____

     Why? _____

6. Which appliance is easier to operate? _____

     Why? _____

7. Which appliance is easier to clean? _____

     Why? _____

8. Which appliance would be easier to store?_____

     Why? _____

9. Which appliance would you rather own?_____

     Why? _____

10. Do you think it would be worthwhile to own both appliances?_____

     Why or why not?_____

Kitchen Utensils

Small Equipment Identification

Activity A   Name _____

Chapter 9   Date _____ Period _____

Identify the name and type (measuring tool, mixing tool, baking tool, thermometer, cutting tool, or other preparation tool) and describe the uses of each of the following pieces of small equipment. Then place a check in the box beside each item that you have in your lab kitchen.

1. ☐

Name: _____

Type: _____

Uses: _____

_____

2. ☐

Name: _____

Type: _____

Uses: _____

_____

3. ☐

Name: _____

Type: _____

Uses: _____

_____

4. ☐

Name: _____

Type: _____

Uses: _____

_____

5. ☐

Name: _____

Type: _____

Uses: _____

_____

(Continued)

Name _____

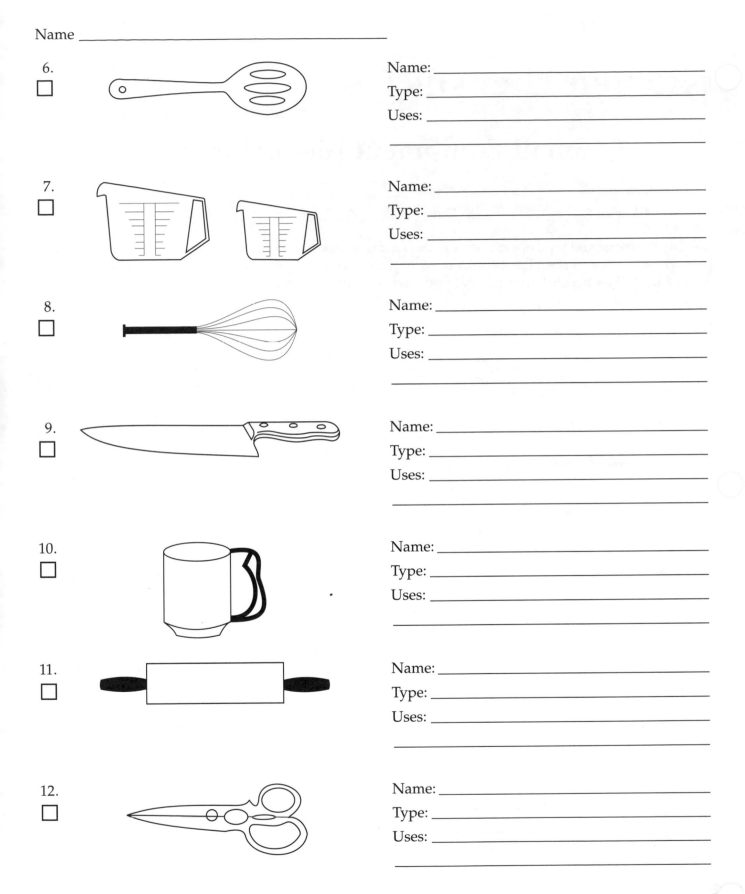

6. ☐

Name: _____

Type: _____

Uses: _____

_____

7. ☐

Name: _____

Type: _____

Uses: _____

_____

8. ☐

Name: _____

Type: _____

Uses: _____

_____

9. ☐

Name: _____

Type: _____

Uses: _____

_____

10. ☐

Name: _____

Type: _____

Uses: _____

_____

11. ☐

Name: _____

Type: _____

Uses: _____

_____

12. ☐

Name: _____

Type: _____

Uses: _____

_____

(Continued)

Name _____

13. ☐

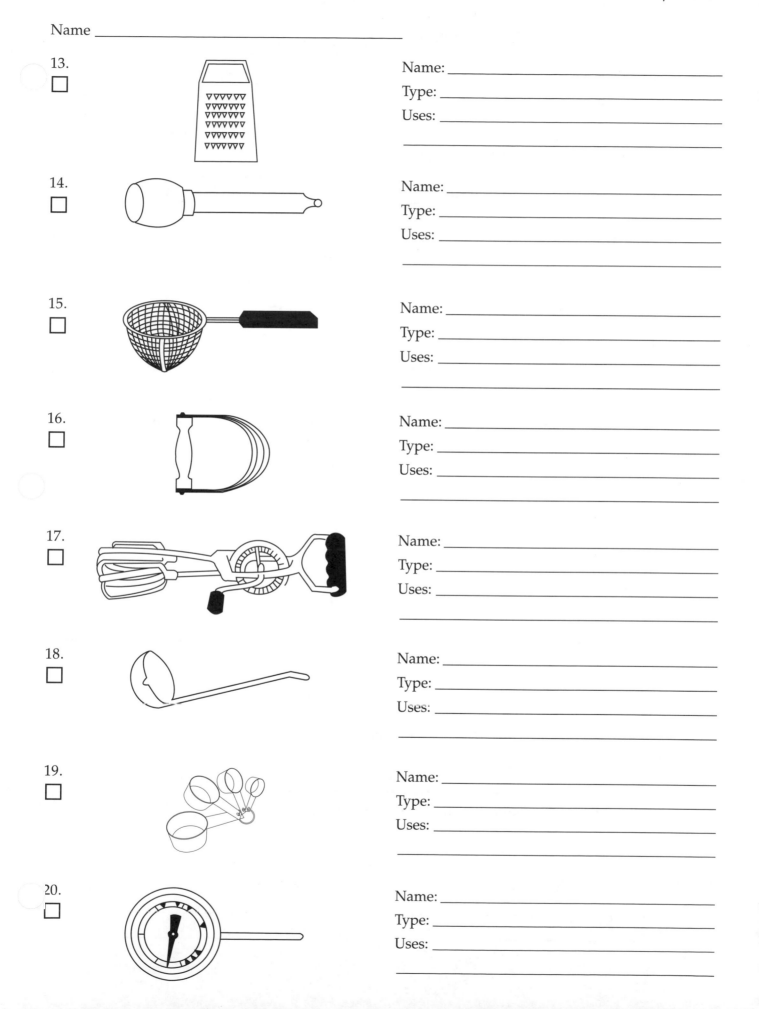

Name: _____

Type: _____

Uses: _____

_____

14. ☐

Name: _____

Type: _____

Uses: _____

_____

15. ☐

Name: _____

Type: _____

Uses: _____

_____

16. ☐

Name: _____

Type: _____

Uses: _____

_____

17. ☐

Name: _____

Type: _____

Uses: _____

_____

18. ☐

Name: _____

Type: _____

Uses: _____

_____

19. ☐

Name: _____

Type: _____

Uses: _____

_____

20. ☐

Name: _____

Type: _____

Uses: _____

_____

Materials Comparison

Activity B

Chapter 9

Name _____

Date _____ Period _____

Complete the chart below by giving the advantages and disadvantages of each of the cookware and bakeware materials listed. Then answer the questions that follow.

Material	Advantages	Disadvantages
Cast iron		
Aluminum		
Copper		
Stainless steel		
Glass		
Glass-ceramic		
Porcelain enamel		
Earthenware		
Plastic		

1. Which material would be your first choice for rangetop cookware? _____

   Why? _____

   _____

2. Which material would be your first choice for conventional bakeware? _____

   Why? _____

   _____

3. Which material would be your first choice for microwave bakeware? _____

   Why? _____

   _____

Microwave Cookware

Activity C   Name _____

Chapter 9   Date _____ Period _____

Explain why each of the following statements about microwave cookware is false.

1. Microwaves should be reflected by microwave cookware.

   _____

   _____

2. Microwaves can pass through metal.

   _____

   _____

3. Metal should never be used in a microwave oven.

   _____

   _____

4. Most people need to buy complete sets of microwave cookware when they purchase microwave ovens.

   _____

   _____

5. Disposable plastic containers from margarine and whipped toppings are recommended for microwave cooking.

   _____

   _____

6. Wooden bowls are a good choice for microwaving liquids.

   _____

   _____

7. Microwave cookware does not get hot so pot holders are not necessary when removing food containers from a microwave oven.

   _____

   _____

8. Square cookware pieces are the best shape for microwave cooking.

   _____

   _____

Equipment Review

Activity D   Name_____

Chapter 9   Date _____ Period _____

Each "clue" below describes a different piece of kitchen equipment. Using these clues, identify the piece of equipment being described.

1. I am preferred by most chefs for incorporating air into foods like souffles and for preventing lumps from forming in sauces.

2. I keep dough from sticking to a rolling pin.

3. I am used to brush butter or sauces on foods.

4. I am several thin, curved pieces of metal attached to a handle, and I am used for making pie crust.

5. I am inserted into the thickest part of meat or poultry to register the internal temperature.

6. I am a four-sided metal tool used to shred and grate foods such as cabbage and cheese.

7. I have a variety of uses including snipping herbs; trimming vegetables; and cutting meat, dough, and pizza.

8. I am used for scraping bowls and saucepans and for folding one ingredient into another.

9. I am used to remove the outer surface of fruits and vegetables.

10. I am made of glass or plastic, and I am used for measuring ingredients such as milk and syrup.

11. I am made of metal or plastic, and I am used for measuring ingredients such as flour and sugar.

12. I am used to measure small amounts of ingredients.

13. I am used to beat, blend, and incorporate air into foods.

14. I am used to roll dough or pastry.

15. I am used to drain fruits, vegetables, and pasta.

16. I am used to cut, slice, and chop foods.

17. I am used to protect countertops when chopping foods.

18. I am used to separate liquid and solid foods.

19. I am used to blend dry ingredients and to remove lumps from flour and powdered sugar.

20. I consist of a small pan that fits into a larger pan, and I am used to cook foods gently.

21. I am used for panbroiling foods or for cooking foods in a small amount of fat.

22. I am a skillet without sides, and I am used for grilling sandwiches and making pancakes.

23. I am a flat sheet made of metal, and I am used for baking cookies.

24. I am an oblong pan with round depressions.

25. I use suction to collect juices from meat and poultry.

1. _____

2. _____

3. _____

4. _____

5. _____

6. _____

7. _____

8. _____

9. _____

10. _____

11. _____

12. _____

13. _____

14. _____

15. _____

16. _____

17. _____

18. _____

19. _____

20. _____

21. _____

22. _____

23. _____

24. _____

25. _____

Planning Meals

Planning for Nutrition

Activity A   Name _____

Chapter 10   Date _____ Period _____

Complete the following statements about planning nutritious meals by using the terms below to fill in the blanks.

appetizer	nutrients	protein
breakfast	lunch	one-dish meals
calories (kilojoules)	Food Guide Pyramid	meal managers
vitamin C	meal patterns	dinner
leftovers	preparation methods	snacks

1. Outlines used for meal planning that are built around the basic foods that are normally served at each meal are called _____.

2. When used together, the _____ and meal patterns can serve as a framework for planning nutritious meals.

3. A good _____ provides energy and helps to prevent a midmorning slump.

4. A good source of _____, usually in the form of fruit or fruit juice, is often included at breakfast.

5. Soups, sandwiches, salads, and casseroles are examples of foods that are often eaten for _____.

6. For many people, _____ is the one meal of the day that can be eaten leisurely and shared with family members.

7. Dinner is often a heavier meal than lunch, and it is usually the richest meal in terms of _____.

8. New England boiled dinner, tuna noodle casserole, and pizza are examples of _____.

9. If the meal manager plans ahead, between-meal _____ can satisfy nutritional needs as well as hunger.

10. When planning meals for people who need to watch their weight, plan foods that are nutritious and low in _____.

11. A light _____, such as tomato juice, is often served as a first course at dinner.

12. _____ can be sure each family member's nutritional needs are met by planning meals for the entire day at one time.

13. For good health, the foods people eat must supply their bodies with certain essential _____.

14. Varying _____ is a way to add variety to meals.

15. Meal managers can often make use of _____ in nutritious luncheon salads, casseroles,

Planned Spending

Activity B   Name _____

Chapter 10   Date _____ Period _____

Read the following statements about planned spending. Circle *T* if the statement is true or *F* if the statement is false.

T   F   1. On the average, families in the United States spend about 50 percent of their income for food.

T   F   2. It costs more to feed a teenager than it does to feed a senior citizen.

T   F   3. All families with similar food needs spend the same amount of money on food.

T   F   4. As family income increases, the use of staple foods, such as beans and rice, tends to increase.

T   F   5. Being able to recognize seasonal food values and choose quality meats and produce are important meal management skills.

T   F   6. A meal manager's available time and energy affect the family food budget.

T   F   7. A family that eats casseroles and canned goods will likely spend more on food than a family that eats steaks and fresh produce.

T   F   8. A family's value system does not affect spending.

T   F   9. A meal manager is responsible for staying within the family's household spending plan when buying food.

T   F   10. A budget is a plan for managing how money is spent.

T   F   11. Money received as tips, gifts, and interest should usually not be included as sources of income in a budget.

T   F   12. Savings should be listed on a budget as a flexible expense.

T   F   13. Food and utility bills are examples of fixed expenses.

T   F   14. Flexible expenses are easier to adjust than fixed expenses.

T   F   15. Protein foods are the most costly group of foods.

T   F   16. During off seasons, canned and frozen fruits and vegetables are usually cheaper than fresh produce.

T   F   17. Small packages of food products are usually better buys than large packages.

T   F   18. A meal manager may be able to save money by preparing more foods from scratch.

T   F   19. Restaurants, concession stands, and vending machines take a portion of a family's food dollar.

T   F   20. Overspending the food budget to stock up on sale items one week may enable a meal manager to underspend the next week.

Planning Satisfying Menus

Activity C   Name _____

Chapter 10   Date _____ Period _____

In the box below, create an illustration of a satisfying meal by either drawing various foods or clipping pictures from a magazine and mounting them. Then evaluate the meal by describing the variety it includes for each of the listed aspects of appetite appeal.

variety of flavors _____

variety of colors _____

variety of textures _____

variety of shapes _____

variety of sizes _____

variety of temperatures _____

Menu

_____

_____

_____

_____

_____

Convenience Comparison

Activity D

Chapter 10

Name _____

Date _____ Period _____

Choose a food that is available in both semiprepared and finished convenience forms. Find a recipe for making this food and attach it to this page. Prepare the two convenience forms and the homemade form of this food and complete the chart below. Then answer the questions that follow.

Semiprepared		Homemade	
Ingredients Cost		Ingredients Cost	
_____ $_____		_____ $_____	
_____ _____		_____ _____	
_____ _____		_____ _____	
_____ +_____		_____ _____	
Product cost $_____		_____ _____	
Preparation time (in minutes) _____		_____ _____	
Minimum wage per minute × .07		_____ _____	
Labor cost +_____		_____ _____	
Total cost $_____		_____ _____	
Finished		_____ +_____	
Product cost $_____		Product cost $_____	
Preparation time (in minutes) _____		Preparation time (in minutes) _____	
Minimum wage per minute × .07		Minimum wage per minute × .07	
Labor cost +_____		Labor cost +_____	
Total cost $_____		Total cost $_____	

	Total Cost	÷	No. of Servings	=	Cost per Serving
A. Semiprepared	_____	÷	_____	=	_____
B. Finished	_____	÷	_____	=	_____
C. Homemade	_____	÷	_____	=	_____

1. How do the preparation times for the three products compare? _____

2. How does the cost preserving for each of the three products compare? _____

3. How do the appearance and flavor of the convenience products compare with those of the homemade product? _____

4. Which product would you prefer to eat? _____

   Why? _____

5. Which product would you prefer to make? _____

   Why? _____

6. When might you use the other forms of this food? _____

   _____

The Smart Consumer

Types of Stores

Activity A

Chapter 11

Name_____

Date_____ Period _____

Complete the chart below by describing the different types of food stores and listing the advantages and disadvantages of each. Then answer the questions that follow.

Type of Store	Description	Advantages	Disadvantages
Supermarket			
Discount supermarket			
Twenty-four hour convience store			
Specialty store			
Delicatessen			
Farmers' market			
Roadside stand			

In which type of store would you prefer to shop? _____

Why?_____

When might you choose to shop in other types of food stores?_____

_____

Shopping for Food

Activity B

Name _____

Chapter 11

Date _____ Period _____

Complete the following statements about shopping for food. Then arrange the circled letters to spell a term related to shopping for food.

1. ○_ _ _ _ _ _ _ _ are substances that are added to food for a specific purpose.

2. Carotene and ultramarine blue are additives used to enhance the _○_ _ _ of foods.

3. Customers may pay higher prices because of the increased cost of longer business hours at 24-hour _ _ _ _ _○_ _ _ _ stores.

4. Be sure to note expiration dates and redemption requirements before using _ _ _ _○_ _ to save money on grocery purchases.

5. A _ _ _ _○_ _ _ _ _ _ _ is a type of store that sells ready-to-eat foods like cold meats and salads.

6. _○_ _ _ _ _ _ supermarkets sell food at reduced prices and in large quantities.

7. _ _○_ _ _ _ markets are a type of store at which food is sold directly from the farm to the consumer.

8. A brand sold only by a store or chain of stores is called a○_ _ _ _ _ _ _ _ _.

9. Making an unplanned purchase without much thought is called _ _ _ _ _○_ _ _ _ _ _ _.

10. A brand that is advertised and sold throughout the country is called a _ _ _ _ _ _○_ _ _ _ _ _ _.

11. Additives like thiamin and niacin are used to add _ _ _ _ _ _○_ _ to foods.

12. _ _○_ _ _ _ foods are foods that have been grown in soil enriched with organic fertilizers and without the use of pesticides.

13. Organically grown foods that have not been treated with preservatives, hormones, antibiotics, or synthetic additives are called _ _ _ _ _ _ _ _ _ _ _ _ ○_ _ _ _ _ _ _ _ foods.

14. Emulsifiers and stabilizers are two types of additives used to aid _ _○_ _ _ _ _ _ _ _.

15. A type of store found near farms during the growing season is a _ _ _ _ _○_ _ _ _ _ _ _ _.

16. A _ _ _○_ _ _ _ _ _ _ _ can help consumers save time, avoid extra trips for forgotten items, and stick to their food budget.

17. Dairies, bakeries, and butcher shops are examples of _○_ _ _ _ _ _ _ stores.

18. Self-service stores that carry both food and nonfood items are _ _ _ _ _○_ _ _ _ _ _.

Circled letters _____

_ _ _ _ _ _ _ _ _ _ _ _ _ _ _ _ _ _ involves evaluating different brands, sizes, and forms of a product before making a purchase decision.

Using Food Advertisements

Activity C   Name _____

Chapter 11   Date _____ Period _____

Use the advertising flyer from a local grocery store to make a shopping list. Use the guide on the left to list the various specials according to the area of the store where you will find them. Then plan balanced meals around the advertised specials in the spaces provided on the right.

Shopping List

Produce
_____
_____
_____

Dairy
_____
_____
_____

Deli
_____
_____
_____

Meat
_____
_____
_____

Canned/packaged foods
_____
_____
_____

Bakery
_____
_____
_____

Frozen foods
_____
_____
_____

Miscellaneous
_____
_____
_____

Breakfast
_____
_____
_____
_____

Lunch
_____
_____
_____
_____

Dinner
_____
_____
_____
_____

Snacks
_____
_____
_____
_____

Reading a Nutrition Label

Activity D

Chapter 11

Name _____

Date _____ Period _____

Answer the questions below about the nutrition label shown.

Nutrition Facts

Serving Size 1/2 cup (228g)
Servings Per Container 1

Amount Per Serving

Calories 230   Calories from Fat 18

% Daily Value*

Total Fat 2g	**3%**
Saturated Fat 2g	**10%**
Cholesterol 10mg	**3%**
Sodium 133mg	**6%**
Total Carbohydrate 43g	**14%**
Dietary Fiber 0g	**0%**
Sugars 28g	
Protein 10g	

Vitamin A 2%	•	Vitamin C 3%	
Calcium 35%	•	Iron 1%	

* Percent Daily Values are based on a 2,000 calorie diet. Your daily values may be higher or lower depending on your calorie needs:

	Calories	2,000	2,500
Total Fat	Less than	65g	80g
Sat Fat	Less than	20g	25g
Cholesterol	Less than	300mg	300mg
Sodium	Less than	2,400mg	2,400mg
Total Carbohydrate		300g	375g
Fiber		25g	30g

Calories per gram:
Fat 9   •   Carbohydrates 4   •   Protein 4

1. What is the size of a serving of this product? _____

   _____

2. How many calories does a serving of this food provide?

   _____

3. How many grams of total fat does this product supply?

   _____

4. What percent of the Daily Value for saturated fat does a serving of this food provide? _____

   _____

5. What is the unit used to measure cholesterol in food products? _____

   _____

6. What is the Daily Value for sodium? _____

7. In a serving of this product, how many calories come from carbohydrate? _____

   _____

8. How much of the carbohydrate in a serving of this product does *not* come from sugars? _____

   _____

9. How much protein does a serving of this product provide? _____

10. What percent of the Daily Value for vitamin C does a serving of this product provide? _____

11. Is this product a better source of calcium or iron? Explain your answer. _____

    _____

12. How many servings of this food would someone on a 2,000 diet need to eat to meet the full Daily Value for total carbohydrate? _____

13. How much fiber does a person on a 2,500 calorie diet need each day? _____

14. How many calories are supplied by a gram of fat? _____

15. What are two items that federal law requires on food labels besides nutrition information? _____

    _____

    _____

Help for Consumers

Activity E   Name_____

Chapter 11   Date _____ Period _____

Complete the following exercises about some of the resources consumers can use to help them receive the most value from their food dollars.

Open Dating

Match the following types of open dating with their definitions. Then give an example of a food product on which each type of date might be found.

_____ 1. pack date

Product:_____

_____ 2. pull (or sell) date

Product:_____

_____ 3. expiration date

Product:_____

_____ 4. freshness date

Product:_____

A. The last day a consumer should use or eat a food.

B. The day the food was manufactured or processed and packaged.

C. The last day a store should sell a product.

D. The last day a product will be at peak quality.

Unit Pricing

The chart below shows the unit price in cents per ounce (28 g) of various brands, forms, and sizes of orange juice. Use the chart to answer the questions that follow about unit pricing.

Fresh	House Brand	National Brand	Generic Brand
32 ounces (1 liter)	N/A *	5.2	N/A
64 ounces (2 liters)	3.4	3.8	

Canned			
6 ounces (188 mL)	5.5	8.2	N/A
46 ounces (1.4 liters)	5.4		4.6

Frozen**			
6 ounces, makes 24 ounces (750 mL)	12.5 (3.1)	15.0 (3.8)	N/A
12 ounces, makes 48 ounces (1.5 liters)	10.4 (2.6)	14.9 (3.7)	9.3 (2.3)
16 ounces, makes 64 ounces (2 L)	9.9 (2.5)	13.0 (3.3)	N/A

* N/A indicates that product is not available.
** Prices in parentheses indicate cost per ounce when reconstituted.

5. What is the most economical brand, form, and size of orange juice overall?_____

6. Which brand and form is the most economical if you want 64 ounces (2 liters) of juice? _____

7. Which form of the house brand is most economical? _____

8. Which size of the national brand of frozen juice is most economical?_____

9. Which size of the house brand of frozen juice is least economical? _____

(Continued)

Name _____

Generic Products
Answer the following questions about generic products.

10. List four kinds of products that are available as generic products. _____
_____

11. What information can be found on generic labels? _____
_____
_____

12. On the average, how much can consumers save over national brands by purchasing generic
products? _____
_____

How much can they save over house brands? _____

13. How might the quality of generic products differ from that of brand name items? _____
_____
_____

14. When might generic products not be a good choice? _____
_____
_____

Universal Product Code
Fill in the blanks to indicate what the corresponding parts of the universal product code identify.

15. _____

16. _____

17. _____

Sources of Consumer Information
18. Complete the chart below by listing and describing three of the sources of consumer information
discussed in the chapter. Then give an example of a consumer problem that each source might help
you solve.

Source	Description	Problem

Getting Started in the Kitchen

Reading a Recipe

Activity A

Chapter 12

Name _____

Date _____ Period _____

Use the recipe below to answer the questions that follow.

Vegetable Pasta Soup
Makes 10 servings

1 c. chopped onion	1 t. basil
2 T. olive oil	1 c. cubed zucchini
1 c. diced carrot	2 16 oz. cans tomatoes
1 c. minced celery	3 c. water
1 t. salt	1 16 oz. can great northern beans, drained
1 t. oregano	¾ c. uncooked pasta
¼ t. pepper	¼ c. chopped fresh parsley

1. In a soup kettle, sauté onions in olive oil until they are soft, about 5 minutes.
2. Add carrot, celery, salt, oregano, pepper, and basil. Cover and cook over low heat for 5 minutes.
3. Stir in zucchini, tomatoes, water, and beans. Cover and simmer gently for 30 minutes.
4. Heat soup to a boil.
5. Add pasta and boil until tender, about 10 minutes.
6. Stir in parsley and serve.

1. List five pieces of equipment you would need to prepare this recipe. _____

   _____

2. What do you need to do to the beans to get them ready to use? _____

3. What do the abbreviations used with each of the following ingredients mean?

   A. onion _____   C. salt _____

   B. olive oil _____   D. tomatoes _____

4. Explain how the onions are to be cut. _____

5. Explain how the carrots are to be cut. _____

6. Explain how the celery is to be cut. _____

7. Explain how the zucchini is to be cut. _____

8. Explain how the onions are to be cooked. _____

9. Explain the cooking term used in step 3. _____

10. Explain the cooking term used in steps 4 and 5. _____

11. If you figure that it would take 10 minutes to wash and cut all the vegetables, how much time would it take to prepare this recipe? _____

12. What is the yield of this recipe? _____

Microwave Cooking

Activity B　　　　　Name _____

Chapter 12　　　　　Date _____ Period _____

Read the following case studies about microwave cooking problems and answer the questions that follow.

1. Carl put a frozen burrito in the microwave oven for 1½ minutes. The burrito was steaming when Carl took it out of the oven and he burned his tongue on the first bite. When Carl cut into the middle of the burrito, however, there were still ice crystals in the center. Why wasn't Carl's burrito hot all the way through? _____

_____

_____

How could Carl have helped the burrito heat more evenly?_____

_____

_____

2. Jason's mother told him a medium-sized potato could be baked in the microwave oven in four minutes. When Jason cooked a potato for four minutes and then cut into it, it was raw in the center. What did Jason's mother forget to mention about microwaving potatoes that kept his from being fully cooked?

_____

_____

_____

3. Stephanie baked some brownies in the microwave oven in a square glass baking dish. When she cut the brownies, Stephanie discovered that the ones in the middle of the pan were moist and chewy. However, the ones in the corners were hard and dry. What caused Stephanie's brownies to be hard in the corners? _____

_____

_____

How could she have prevented this from happening?_____

_____

_____

4. Manuel tightly covered a vegetable tray with plastic wrap before putting it in the microwave oven. Two minutes later he looked through the window of the oven door. Manuel was surprised to see that the wrap had formed a huge bubble over the tray. What caused the plastic wrap to form a bubble and how could this be prevented?_____

_____

_____

How should Manuel remove the wrap to avoid getting burned? _____

_____

_____

Changing Recipe Yield

Activity C   Name _____

Chapter 12   Date _____ Period _____

In the spaces provided, write the yield and amounts of ingredients for a half recipe and a double recipe. Keep all measurements in the same units shown in the recipe. Then answer the questions that follow.

Half Recipe	Turkey Joes	Double Recipe
1. _____	Serves 6 to 8	11. _____
2. _____	1½ pounds ground turkey	12. _____
3. _____	½ cup chopped onion	13. _____
4. _____	1 tablespoon flour	14. _____
5. _____	2 teaspoons brown sugar	15. _____
6. _____	1 teaspoon ground mustard	16. _____
7. _____	1½ teaspoons chili powder	17. _____
8. _____	⅓ cup water	18. _____
9. _____	2 tablespoons cider vinegar	19. _____
10. _____	1½ cups chili sauce	20. _____

21. How would you measure the amount of flour needed for half a recipe? _____

22. How would you measure the amount of water needed for half a recipe? _____

23. Convert the amount of brown sugar needed for a double recipe into units that would require the least amount of measuring. _____

24. Convert the amount of chili powder needed for a double recipe into units that would require the least amount of measuring. _____

25. Convert the amount of vinegar needed for a double recipe into units that would require the least amount of measuring. _____

26. What is the metric equivalent of the amount of onion needed for half a recipe? _____

27. What is the metric equivalent of the amount of mustard needed for half a recipe? _____

28. What is the metric equivalent of the amount of vinegar needed for half a recipe? _____

29. What is the metric equivalent of the amount of chili sauce needed for half a recipe? _____

30. What is the metric equivalent of the amount of mustard needed for a single recipe? _____

31. What is the metric equivalent of the amount of water needed for a single recipe? _____

32. What is the metric equivalent of the amount of onion needed for a double recipe? _____

33. What is the metric equivalent of the amount of water needed for a double recipe? _____

34. What is the metric equivalent of the amount of vinegar needed for a double recipe? _____

Making a Time-Work Schedule

Activity D   Name_____

Chapter 12   Date _____ Period _____

Plan a menu for a nutritious meal and make a time-work schedule for preparing it by following these steps:

1. List your menu items in the first column of the Preparation Task Chart.

2. Fill in your estimates for the time required for preparing, cooking, and serving each menu item.

3. Add the total time required to prepare each item.

4. In the last column of the chart, rank the menu items in order of the total time required to prepare them, with 1 requiring the most time.

5. Use the information in the Preparation Task Chart to complete the Time-Work Schedule. List the most important preparation tasks and specific times for completing them. Remember to allow your schedule to be flexible.

Preparation Task Chart

Menu	Preparation Time	Cooking Time	Serving Time	Total Time	Rank
Table setting			10	10	

Time-Work Schedule

Time	Tasks

Meat

Meat Inspection and Grading

Activity A

Chapter 13

Name_____

Date _____ Period _____

Answer the following questions related to meat inspection and grading.

1. When must meat be federally inspected? _____

2. What does an inspection stamp on a wholesale cut indicate about the meat?_____

_____

3. What is the difference between a yield grade and a quality grade?_____

_____

_____

4. Who oversees the voluntary meat grading program?_____

In each of the following pairs of characteristics of beef, choose the letter of the one that would receive the higher quality grade.

5. _____ A. less marbling
    B. more marbling

6. _____ A. younger animal
    B. older animal

7. _____ A. fine muscle texture
    B. course muscle texture

8. What are the eight beef quality grades? _____

_____

9. Which of the top three grades of beef usually costs less?_____

10. Which of the top three grades of beef do hotels and restaurants usually buy? _____

11. How are the lower grades of beef often used?_____

12. What are the six quality grades for veal? _____

_____

13. What are the two quality grades for pork?_____

14. What are the five quality grades for lamb?_____

_____

15. Which veal, pork, and lamb carcasses are likely to receive the highest quality grades?_____

_____

Selection and Storage of Meats

Activity B   Name _____

Chapter 13   Date _____ Period _____

Determine what terms related to selecting and storing meats are missing from the statements. Write the terms in the blanks at the right.

1. The edible portion of mammals is called _____.   1. _____

2. Mature cattle over 12 months of age are called _____.   2. _____

3. Animal carcasses are divided into smaller pieces called _____ for easier handling by meat cutters.   3. _____

4. At the grocery store, meat cutters divide meats into smaller pieces called _____.   4. _____

5. A ground beef product that can have extra fat added to it during grinding is called _____.   5. _____

6. Very young beef is called _____.   6. _____

7. The meat of swine is called _____.   7. _____

8. Smoked pork belly meat is known as _____.   8. _____

9. The meat of sheep less than one year old is sold as _____.   9. _____

10. The meat from sheep over two years of age is called _____.   10. _____

11. The edible parts of an animal other than the muscles are called _____.   11. _____

12. The stomach lining of beef is a popular meat product called _____.   12. _____

13. A round, purple inspection stamp assures buyers of wholesale cuts that the meat is _____.   13. _____

14. Flecks of fat throughout the lean of meat are known as _____.   14. _____

15. The USDA _____ shield assures consumers that meat has met certain standards of quality.   15. _____

16. _____ shape can help consumers identify whether a meat cut comes from a tender part of an animal.   16. _____

17. T-shaped bones are found in _____ cuts of meat.   17. _____

18. Muscles receiving little _____ produce the most tender cuts of meat.   18. _____

19. To help consumers with meat selection, most retail stores follow a labeling system developed under the _____ program.   19. _____

20. Meat _____ like dried beans and rice can help stretch meat dollars.   20. _____

Cooking by Cut

Activity C   Name _____

Chapter 13   Date _____ Period _____

Look at the location in the animal of the following beef wholesale cuts. Write *T* in the blank if the cut is tender. Write *LT* in the blank if the cut is less tender. (You may want to refer to Chart 13-1 on page 237 of the text.

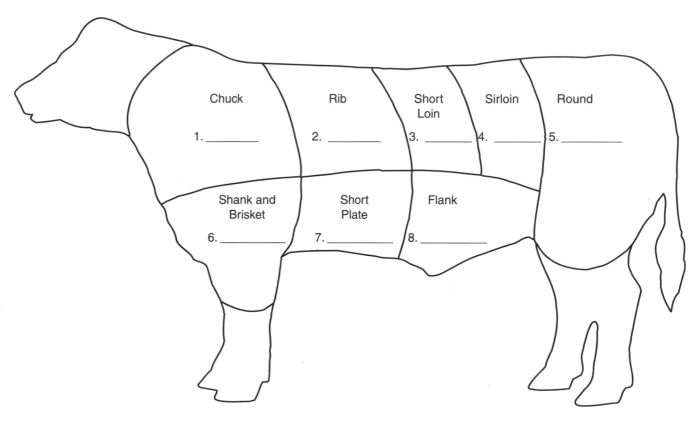

9. List the four dry cooking methods.

_____

_____

_____

_____

10. List the two moist cooking methods.

_____

_____

Read the following list of retail cuts of beef. Place a *D* in the blank if a cut should be cooked with dry heat. Place an *M* in the blank if a cut should be cooked with moist heat. Place an *E* in the blank if a cut can be cooked with either type of heat.

_____ 11. brisket

_____ 12. ground beef

_____ 13. sirloin steak

_____ 14. short ribs

_____ 15. arm pot roast

_____ 16. round steak

_____ 17. T-bone steak

_____ 18. rib roast

_____ 19. rump roast

_____ 20. flank steak

Meat Cookery Methods

Activity D   Name_____

Chapter 13   Date _____ Period _____

Match each of the following statements with the meat cooking method it describes by placing the correct letter in the space provided. Then answer the questions that follow.

_____ 1. Place meat with the fat side up on a rack in a large, shallow pan. Meat is cooked, uncovered, in a slow oven until it reaches the desired degree of doneness.

_____ 2. Meat is cooked under a direct flame or under a direct heating element.

_____ 3. Meat is cooked, uncovered, in a heavy skillet or griddle without using fat.

_____ 4. Meat is cooked in a small amount of fat or in deep fat.

_____ 5. Meat is browned slowly, and then it is cooked in a small amount of liquid over low heat.

_____ 6. Meat is covered with water or stock. The kettle is covered, and the meat is allowed to simmer until it is tender.

A. braising

B. broiling

C. cooking in liquid

D. frying

E. microwaving

F. panbroiling

G. roasting

7. What are the recommended time frames during which refrigerated meats should be cooked or frozen?

_____

_____

8. What are the food safety guidelines regarding marinade used for raw meat?_____

_____

9. What types of variety meats may be cooked by dry heat?_____

_____

10. How should meat be thawed? _____

_____

11. Why is it recommended that meat not be thawed on the kitchen counter? _____

_____

12. A frozen roast would require approximately _____ percent more time to cook than a thawed roast.

13. When broiling frozen meats, why should you place the meat farther away from the heat source than you would place thawed meats? _____

_____

14. Why should meats be covered when they are cooked in a microwave oven? _____

_____

15. What type of meat cuts work best for microwave cooking? _____

_____

16. What type of meat cuts will brown naturally in a microwave oven?_____

_____

Poultry

Poultry Pointers

Activity A

Chapter 14

Name _____

Date _____ Period _____

Fill in the puzzle with the words needed to complete the tips on poultry selection and storage given below.

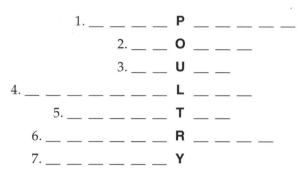

1. __ __ __ __ **P** __ __ __ __ __

2. __ __ **O** __ __ __

3. __ __ **U** __ __

4. __ __ __ __ __ __ __ **L** __ __ __

5. __ __ __ __ __ **T** __ __

6. __ __ __ __ __ __ **R** __ __ __ __

7. __ __ __ __ __ __ **Y**

1. Poultry is a good source of _____, iron, thiamin, riboflavin, and niacin.

2. Poultry can be purchased fresh-chilled or _____.

3. Most poultry is marketed _____, so the meat is tender and suitable for all cooking methods.

4. Proper storage of poultry is important to inhibit the growth of _____, an illness-causing bacteria.

5. Any domesticated bird is called _____.

6. When buying poultry, beware of pale, dry, frosty areas that indicate _____. (Two words.)

7. Poultry may be graded voluntarily for _____.

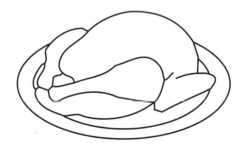

Poultry Selection and Storage

Activity B   Name _____

Chapter 14   Date _____ Period _____

Write the letter of the answer that best completes each statement in the space provided.

_____ 1. Dark meat is slightly _____ in fat than light meat.
  A. lower
  B. higher

_____ 2. A lot of the fat in poultry is located _____.
  A. throughout the muscle
  B. just under the skin

_____ 3. All poultry sold in interstate commerce must be federally _____ for wholesomeness.
  A. inspected
  B. graded

_____ 4. Chicken breasts, legs, and thighs are _____ than wings and backs.
  A. meatier
  B. less meaty

_____ 5. Poultry contains _____ bone in relation to muscle than does red meat.
  A. more
  B. less

_____ 6. You need to allow about _____ per serving when buying chicken.
  A. ½ pound
  B. ¾ pound

_____ 7. Dark meat has a _____ flavor than light meat.
  A. milder
  B. stronger

_____ 8. Ducks and geese have _____ meat.
  A. both light and dark
  B. all dark

_____ 9. Ducks and geese have _____ fat than chickens or turkeys.
  A. more
  B. less

_____ 10. Canned poultry items are generally _____ expensive than fresh-chilled or frozen poultry.
  A. more
  B. less

_____ 11. Poultry parts are _____ perishable than whole birds.
  A. more
  B. less

_____ 12. Wrap and store giblets _____ the rest of the bird.
  A. separately from
  B. with

_____ 13. Poultry can be stored in the freezer for _____.
  A. six to eight months
  B. up to one year

_____ 14. Frozen poultry that has thawed _____ be refrozen
  A. can
  B. should not

Poultry Cookery

Activity C   Name _____

Chapter 14   Date _____ Period _____

Answer the following questions about poultry cookery.

1. What are the principles for cooking poultry and what happens when they are not followed? _____

    _____

    _____

    _____

2. If you do not have a meat thermometer, how can you tell if poultry is cooked? _____

    _____

    _____

    _____

3. List the dry heat methods often used for cooking poultry.

    List the moist heat methods often used for cooking poultry.

    _____

    _____

    _____

    _____

4. Why should roasted poultry stand 10 to 15 minutes before it is carved? _____

    _____

5. What does trussing a bird accomplish? _____

    _____

    _____

6. If a bird is to be stuffed, when should this be done? Why? _____

    _____

    _____

7. What temperature should stuffing packed into the cavity of a bird reach? _____

8. How can you prevent the breast of a large bird from overbrowning? _____

    _____

    _____

9. How do cooking bags shorten cooking time? _____

    _____

10. How far from the heat source should poultry be broiled? _____

11. How long will it take chicken to broil? _____

(Continued)

Name _____

12. How is poultry prepared for frying? _____

_____

_____

13. How deep should the fat be for frying chicken? _____

14. What is another name for oven-frying? _____

15. How can you help braised poultry develop a crisp crust? _____

_____

16. What ingredients can be added to flavor poultry during stewing? _____

17. How might stewed poultry be used? _____

_____

18. List three benefits of using a microwave oven for preparing poultry. _____

_____

_____

19. How should drumsticks be arranged to ensure even cooking in a microwave oven? _____

_____

_____

20. When should you thaw frozen poultry? _____

21. How can frozen poultry be thawed quickly? _____

_____

_____

22. What is the advantage of boning chicken yourself? _____

Fish and Shellfish

Selecting Fish and Shellfish

Activity A

Chapter 15

Name _____

Date _____ Period _____

Complete the chart below by defining the characteristics that identify the different classes of finfish and shellfish. Then list each of the following water animals in the appropriate section of this chart. (Hint: Read the chapter information on cooking methods as well as the information on classification before completing this activity.)

catfish	flounder	mackerel	scallops
clams	haddock	oysters	shrimp
cod	halibut	red snapper	swordfish
crabs	lobster	salmon	trout

Finfish	
Lean fish:	Fat fish:
Examples:	Examples:

Shellfish	
Mollusks:	Crustaceans:
Examples:	Examples:

(Continued)

Name _____

Identify the following forms in which fresh finfish can be purchased.

1. _____

2. _____

3. _____

4. _____

5. _____

Match each of the following statements about shellfish with the animal it describes by placing the correct letter in the space provided.

_____ 6. When purchased fresh, this animal's shell should be tightly closed or should close when you touch it.

_____ 7. When purchased shucked, this animal should be plump, creamy in color, and odorless.

_____ 8. The bay variety of this animal is small and creamy white or pink. The deep sea variety is larger and white.

_____ 9. Blue and Dungeness are the most common species of this animal sold in the United States.

_____ 10. The shell covering this animal should be firmly attached and the animal should be odorless.

_____ 11. When this animal is alive, its tail should snap back quickly after it is flattened.

A. shrimp

B. oysters

C. crabs

D. lobster

E. clams

F. scallops

Finfish Cookery

Activity B   Name _____

Chapter 15   Date _____ Period _____

Read the definitions and look at the scrambled letters. Then write the correct terms in the blanks.

1. Refers to cooking in a simmering liquid.   GIPHANOC _ _ _ _ _ _ _ _

2. Involves cooking steaks, fillets, or whole fish under a direct heat source until the fish flakes easily with a fork.   LOIBRING _ _ _ _ _ _ _ _

3. A cooking method used to cook steaks, fillets, or whole fish in the oven.   GABNIK _ _ _ _ _ _

4. A cooking method where fish is placed on a rack over simmering liquid in a tightly covered pan.   MEATSING _ _ _ _ _ _ _ _

5. Involves coating fish with crumbs or batter and then cooking it in fat.   YIFRNG _ _ _ _ _ _

6. A cooking method that requires whole fish to be rotated one-quarter turn several times during the cooking period to ensure even cooking.   WICAMINROVG _ _ _ _ _ _ _ _ _ _ _

7. Which of the cooking methods described above are recommended for cooking fat fish?

_____

_____

8. Which of the cooking methods described above are recommended for cooking lean fish?

_____

_____

9. What general guide can be used to time fish cooked by a variety of cooking methods?

_____

_____

To what two cooking methods does this guide not apply?

_____

10. In the space provided, plan a dinner menu that includes a finfish entree.

_____

_____

_____

_____

_____

Fish Maze

Activity C

Chapter 15

Name _____

Date _____ Period _____

Complete the statements about the selection and storage of fish by filling in the blanks. Then find the terms in the word maze and circle them. (Terms are located horizontally, vertically, and diagonally in the maze.)

```
D  D  N  T  P  O  A  C  H  Z  R  F  A  L  A  I  B  C  D  D
A  R  A  S  E  R  C  S  S  B  I  O  D  O  R  G  P  B  E  E
C  A  E  B  E  S  D  N  Y  L  I  O  R  B  Q  C  P  P  K  V
L  W  L  S  X  D  H  A  L  A  R  F  E  S  T  E  A  M  C  E
T  N  R  E  S  C  T  E  E  Q  U  A  G  T  R  L  R  F  U  I
Q  I  K  W  X  E  T  C  L  O  O  I  T  E  S  O  B  E  H  N
F  A  G  A  J  Z  D  A  Z  L  L  A  Y  R  F  H  O  D  S  E
B  V  M  I  E  U  I  T  Y  L  F  A  H  T  H  W  I  M  Y  D
P  V  U  O  U  T  K  S  N  E  E  I  A  S  C  A  L  L  O  P
U  O  S  D  H  K  S  U  L  L  O  M  S  L  U  O  I  P  J  U
S  H  R  I  M  P  L  R  X  N  I  L  K  H  S  I  F  N  I  F
O  T  I  N  S  P  E  C  T  I  O  N  W  J  V  K  S  M  P  O
W  N  E  E  K  M  R  X  Y  L  N  J  T  L  I  M  R  N  H  N
```

1. Water animals that have both fins and backbones are called _____.

2. Water animals that have shells instead of backbones are called _____.

3. Fish that have very little fat in their flesh are called _____ fish.

4. Fish with fattier flesh are called _____ fish.

5. A shellfish that has a soft body that is partially or fully covered by a hard shell is called a(n) _____.

6. A shellfish that is covered by a crustlike shell and has a segmented body is called a(n) _____.

7. In some parts of the world, people use concentrated fish protein, known as fish _____ to increase the protein level of the diet.

8. Saltwater fish are one of the most important sources of the mineral _____.

1. _____

2. _____

3. _____

4. _____

5. _____

6. _____

7. _____

8. _____

(Continued)

Name _____

9. The National Marine Fisheries Service provides a voluntary _____ program for the fish industry.

9. _____

10. The factors used to determine the quality grade of fish are appearance, flavor, lack of defects, and _____.

10. _____

11. A fish that is marketed as it comes from the water is called a _____ fish.

11. _____

12. A fish that has the entrails removed is a _____ fish.

12. _____

13. A fish that has the entrails, head, fins, and scales removed is a _____ fish.

13. _____

14. A cross-sectional slice taken from a dressed fish is called a(n) _____.

14. _____

15. A side of a fish cut lengthwise away from the backbone is called a(n) _____.

15. _____

16. These crustaceans are marketed according to the number needed to weigh 1 pound (450 g) in sizes such as jumbo, large, and medium.

16. _____

17. Shrimp sold without the intestinal tract are labeled as _____ shrimp.

17. _____

18. Oysters and clams can be purchased removed from the shell, or _____.

18. _____

19. These crustaceans are dark, blue-green when removed from the water.

19. _____

20. These mollusks are available in tiny bay and large deep sea varieties.

20. _____

21. For this method of cooking, fish should be at least 1 inch (2.5 cm) thick.

21. _____

22. Oven temperature should be 400° to 450°F (200° to 230°C) for this method of cooking fish.

22. _____

23. You can use a pan, the oven, or deep fat to cook fish by this method.

23. _____

24. You _____ fish by cooking it in simmering liquid.

24. _____

25. You need little liquid when you _____ fish because the fish cooks inside a covered utensil.

25. _____

26. You _____ live lobster, shrimp, and crab by plunging the shellfish into boiling, salted water until it is partially cooked.

26. _____

Investigating Shellfish

Activity D

Chapter 15

Name _____

Date _____ Period _____

Use library resources, supermarket research, and the form below to write a brief report about one type of shellfish.

Type of shellfish: _____

Part(s) of the body eaten as food: _____

_____

Varieties eaten as food: _____

_____

_____

Waters where they are commonly found: _____

_____

_____

How they are caught: _____

_____

How they are prepared for market: _____

_____

Market forms: _____

Market sizes: _____

Market price range: _____

How they are commonly cooked: _____

_____

Recipe calling for this type of shellfish: _____

Ingredients: _____

_____

_____

_____

Directions: _____

_____

_____

_____

_____

Serves: _____

Eggs

Selection and Storage of Eggs

Activity A

Chapter 16

Name _____

Date _____ Period _____

Complete the following exercises related to the selection and storage of eggs.

Fill-in-the-Blanks: Complete the following statements by filling in the blanks.

1. Regardless of price, most shoppers buy _____ size eggs.

2. Eggs are one of the best food sources of _____.

3. Because egg yolks are high in _____, some experts recommend that people limit the number of egg yolks they eat.

4. Eggs are graded for quality by a system called _____.

5. Grade _____ eggs are the best choice to use when appearance is important, as in poaching or frying.

Identification:

6. From the list below, check the four quality factors that are used to determine egg grades.

_____ A. condition of the shell

_____ B. condition of the yolk

_____ C. size of the air cell

_____ D. color of the shell

_____ E. clearness and thickness of the egg white

_____ F. size of the egg

_____ G. nutrient content

Short Answer: Answer the following questions to show your understanding.

7. What two factors affect variation in egg prices? _____

8. Why are Grade B eggs rarely seen in food stores? _____

9. How are egg sizes determined? _____

_____

10. For what size eggs are recipes usually formulated? _____

11. What causes some eggs to have brown shells? _____

12. How should eggs be stored in the refrigerator? _____

_____

13. How long can eggs be safely stored in a refrigerator? _____

_____

14. How should leftover egg yolks and egg whites be stored?

Yolks: _____

Whites: _____

Functions of Eggs

Activity B   Name _____

Chapter 16   Date _____ Period _____

The main functions performed by eggs in recipes are listed below. Describe these functions and give an example of a food product in which each function is performed.

Function	Description	Food product
Emulsifier		
Foam		
Thickener		
Binding agent		
Interfering agent		
Structure agent		
Nutrient additive		
Flavoring additive		
Coloring agent		

Egg Dishes

Activity C   Name _____

Chapter 16   Date _____ Period _____

Place the specified letter in the blank to indicate whether each of the following statements is true or false. When completed, the letters will spell out a term related to the chapter.

_____   1. Temperature, time, and the addition of other ingredients affect egg coagulation. (E = true; M = false)

_____   2. High temperatures are recommended for egg cookery. (G = true; M = false)

_____   3. Scrambled eggs should be stirred constantly during cooking. (G = true; U = false)

_____   4. When poaching eggs, a small amount of vinegar added to the cooking water will keep the egg whites from spreading. (L = true; C = false)

_____   5. When frying an egg, covering the skillet will cause the upper surface of the egg to cook more quickly. (S = true; O = false)

_____   6. When baking eggs, individual baking dishes should be placed in a shallow casserole filled with 1 inch of warm water. (I = true; O = false)

_____   7. Soft-cooked eggs prepared by the hot water method are boiled in water for one to four minutes. (K = true; F = false)

_____   8. A greenish-colored ring around the yolk of a hard-cooked egg is toxic and should not be eaten. (E = true; Y = false)

_____   9. Egg yolks should be gently punctured before microwaving to prevent them from bursting. (I = true; R = false)

_____   10. When making a puffy omelet, the egg yolks and egg whites are beaten separately and then folded together. (N = true; Y = false)

_____   11. Soufflés should be allowed to stand 10 to 15 minutes after being removed from the oven. (M = true; G = false)

_____   12. Beading is the leakage of liquid from a gel that sometimes occurs between a meringue and a pie filling. (E = true; A = false)

_____   13. Hard meringues contain a lower proportion of sugar than soft meringues. (T = true; G = false)

_____   14. Soft custards usually contain less egg than baked custards. (E = true; H = false)

_____   15. The use of low heat can cause soft custard to curdle. (O = true; N = false)

_____   16. A baked custard is done if the tip of a knife inserted into the center comes out clean. (T = true; D = false)

Scrambled Eggs

Activity D
Chapter 16

Name _____

Date _____ Period _____

Unscramble the letters below. Then use the words to complete the following statements about eggs.

ACNPHIGO   _ _ _ _ _ _ _ _

GFLINOD   _ _ _ _ _ _ _

OESLUFF   _ _ _ _ _ _ _

IWEPEGN   _ _ _ _ _ _ _

CTASUDR   _ _ _ _ _ _ _

GTINFIEERRN NEATG   _ _ _ _ _ _ _ _ _ _ _ _ _ _ _

AIEGBND   _ _ _ _ _ _ _

NOIELSMU   _ _ _ _ _ _ _ _

SSEENSRIY   _ _ _ _ _ _ _ _

DANNCLIG   _ _ _ _ _ _ _ _

SREIRHD   _ _ _ _ _ _ _

NRIUMEGE   _ _ _ _ _ _ _ _

LEEOTM   _ _ _ _ _ _

GUUCLOMA   _ _ _ _ _ _ _ _

FITSF AEKP   _ _ _ _ _ _ _ _ _

1. When egg whites are beaten to the _____ _____ stage, the peaks stand up straight.

2. Eggs act as an _____ _____ in some frozen desserts by inhibiting the formation of large ice crystals.

3. A puffy _____ is baked in a preheated oven.

4. Golden droplets that appear on the surface of a meringue are known as _____.

5. The blending process used to avoid a loss of air when combining egg white foams with other ingredients is known as _____.

6. _____ is done by simmering the egg in water or steaming it in a cup over simmering water.

7. Eggs are used to form a permanent _____ in mayonnaise and hollandaise sauce.

8. Eggs can be scrambled, poached, and _____ in a microwave oven.

9. Custards are baked in a pan of warm water to help prevent _____.

10. A _____ is a light, airy egg dish that can be served as a dessert or a main dish, depending on the added ingredients.

11. The layer of moisture that sometimes forms between a meringue and a pie filling is known as _____.

12. A hard _____ may be used as a dessert base.

13. When heat is applied to eggs, they form a _____, or smooth, thickened mass.

14. The _____ process illuminates the interior structure of eggs so skilled people can identify eggs that do not meet quality standards.

15. A mixture of milk or cream, eggs, sugar, and a flavoring that is cooked until thickened is a _____.

Dairy Products

Dairy Product Variety

Activity A

Chapter 17

Name _____

Date _____ Period _____

Underline the dairy products and foods containing dairy products in the menus below. Write a shopping list of all the dairy products you would need to buy to prepare these menus. Then plan a snack for each day using some of the leftover dairy products.

	Day 1	Day 2
Breakfast	Scrambled Eggs Sausage Links Whole Wheat Toast Grapefruit Half Milk Coffee	Bagels Cream Cheese Orange Juice Chocolate Milk
Lunch	Grilled American Cheese Sandwiches Cream of Tomato Soup Tossed Salad Baked Apple Lemonade	Grilled Ham and Swiss Sandwiches Fruit Salad Yogurt Dressing Sugar Cookies Cola
Dinner	Roast Beef Mashed Potatoes Broccoli Cheddar Cheese Sauce Cloverleaf Rolls Pumpkin Pie Whipped Cream Milk	Broiled Fish Rice Pilaf Sautéed Asparagus Peach Half Cottage Cheese Butter Pecan Ice Cream Iced Tea
Snack		

Shopping List

_____   _____

_____   _____

_____   _____

_____   _____

Cheese Tasting

Activity B   Name _____

Chapter 17   Date _____ Period _____

Sample a variety of cheeses. In the chart below, list the kinds of cheese you sampled and describe their appearance, texture, and flavor.

Kind of Cheese	Appearance	Texture	Flavor

Which of the above cheeses would you recommend for each of the following uses? (Cheeses may be listed under more than one category.)

Appetizers and Snacks	Sandwiches	Cooking	Desserts
_____	_____	_____	_____
_____	_____	_____	_____
_____	_____	_____	_____
_____	_____	_____	_____
_____	_____	_____	_____

Milk Cookery

Activity C   Name _____

Chapter 17   Date _____ Period _____

Undesirable reactions that can occur when cooking with milk are given below. Identify each problem by reading the clues. Then describe a method that could be used to prevent the undesirable reaction.

Problem 1. _____ Clumps have formed in a scalloped potato and ham casserole.	This problem can be prevented by _____ _____ _____
Problem 2. _____ A solid layer has formed on the surface of hot chocolate.	This problem can be prevented by _____ _____ _____
Problem 3. _____ Milk heated in a pan has a brown color and a coating has formed on the bottom of the pan.	This problem can be prevented by _____ _____ _____

The steps for preparing a white sauce are listed below. Read the steps and reorganize them so that they are in the correct order by placing the letters of the corresponding steps in the blanks. When completed, the letters will spell out the name of a white sauce recipe variation that is often combined with meat, fish, or vegetables.

1. _____ S — Allow sauce to reach a boil.

2. _____ A — Slowly add the cold milk, stirring constantly until the sauce is smooth.

3. _____ U — Remove from heat.

4. _____ P — Combine with other foods and serve.

5. _____ E — Stir fat, flour, and seasonings until a smooth paste is formed.

6. _____ O — Cook for one minute longer to thoroughly cook the starch.

7. _____ C — Melt the fat over low heat.

8. _____ M — Cook the sauce over moderate heat, stirring gently.

9. _____ R — Remove the pan from heat and quickly stir in the flour and seasonings.

10. List five uses of white sauce in cooking.

    A. _____

    B. _____

    C. _____

    D. _____

    E. _____

Dairy Products Crossword

Activity D

Chapter 17

Name _____

Date _____ Period _____

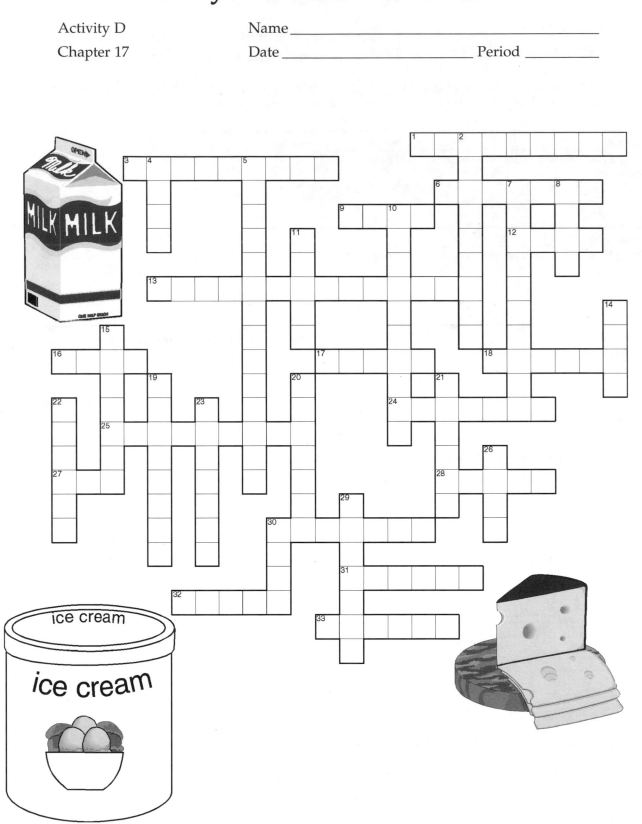

Name _____

Across

1. Special organisms are added to light cream to give it the thick, creamy body and distinct flavor of _____ _____.

3. Burning that results in a color change is _____.

6. _____ cheese products are made from other cheeses.

9. Most of the milk consumed in the United States comes from _____.

12. A _____ is a smooth paste made from flour and melted fat.

13. Heating milk to destroy harmful bacteria is called _____.

16. Most of the fat is removed from nonfat or _____ milk.

17. A gelatin _____ is a milk-based dessert thickened with unflavored gelatin.

18. A rich, thickened cream soup that is often made with shellfish is a _____.

24. A cream soup made with unthickened milk that is often thickened with potatoes is _____.

25. Nutrients have been added in amounts greater than would naturally occur in _____ milk products.

27. _____ processed milk has been heated to a higher temperature than regular pasteurized milk to further increase its shelf life.

28. The milk, yogurt, and cheese group of the Food Guide Pyramid is made up of _____ products.

30. A gummy substance made from the bones and some connective tissue of animals is _____.

31. A concentrated form of milk available in both ripened and unripened varieties is _____.

32. Butter made without salt is called _____ butter.

33. Churning pasteurized and specially cultured sweet or sour cream produces _____.

Down

2. Cheeses that are ready for marketing as soon as the whey has been removed are called _____ cheeses.

4. The solid part of coagulated milk is called _____.

5. A mechanical process that prevents cream from rising to the surface of milk is _____.

7. Heating can cause the lactose in milk to _____, or change to a brown, bitter substance.

8. A solid layer that often forms on the surface of milk during heating is called _____.

10. A thickened milk product made from fat, flour, milk, and seasonings is _____ _____.

11. To _____ foods means to turn them into a thick, smooth liquid with the use of a sieve or blender.

14. The liquid part of coagulated milk is called _____.

15. The fat portion of milk is called _____.

19. _____ is when the proteins in milk coagulate and form clumps due to high temperatures, acids, tannins, enzymes, or salts.

20. Gelatin must be soaked in cold liquid to _____ the granules, causing them to absorb water.

21. The portion of milk containing most of the vitamins, minerals, protein, and sugar is the milk _____.

22. A cultured milk product that may contain added nonfat milk solids and flavorings or fruits is _____.

23. Controlled amounts of bacteria, mold, yeast, or enzymes are used to make _____ cheeses.

26. Whole _____ contains at least 3.25 percent milkfat and 8.25 percent milk solids.

29. Dairy products are a major source of _____ in the diet.

30. In areas where grazing land is scarce, people often use milk from the _____.

Dairy Desserts

Activity E

Chapter 17

Name _____

Date _____ Period _____

Complete the following statements about puddings, gelatin creams, and frozen desserts by filling in the blanks using the terms below.

cornstarch pudding   frozen yogurt

parfaits   tapioca pudding

Bavarian creams   Spanish creams

sherbet   mousses

indian pudding   charlottes

ice cream   bread pudding

1. _____ contains fruit juices, sugar, and milk with beaten egg whites, whipped cream, or gelatin added to improve its texture.

2. _____ are prepared by folding beaten egg whites, whipped cream, and flavorings or fruit purees into a whipped, thickened gelatin.

3. _____ contains milk and eggs that form a custard around bread cubes.

4. _____ are prepared by adding a large amount of whipped cream to a Bavarian cream and pouring the mixture into a mold lined with ladyfingers.

5. _____ contains milk, cornmeal, eggs, salt, and molasses.

6. _____ is made from milk, cream, sugar, and flavoring, and it is stirred during the freezing process to produce a creamy texture.

7. _____ is made from a mixture of active yogurt cultures, sugar, stabilizer, nonfat solids, and flavorings.

8. _____ are prepared by pouring a sugar syrup over beaten eggs, then folding whipped cream into the egg mixture and adding a flavoring. They are frozen without stirring.

9. _____ is made with milk, cornstarch, sugar, salt, and flavoring, and it is cooked until thickened.

10. _____ contain sweetened and flavored whipped cream and are frozen without stirring.

11. _____ contains milk, tapioca, sugar, salt, eggs, and flavoring.

12. _____ are prepared by adding unflavored gelatin to a stirred custard while the custard is warm.

Fruits

Fruit Scramble

Activity A   Name _____

Chapter 18   Date _____ Period _____

Unscramble the following letters to spell out the names of fruits. Then check the appropriate column to identify the classification of each fruit.

Fruits	Berries	Drupes	Pomes	Citrus Fruits	Melons	Tropical Fruits
1. ganrose =						
2. palpes =						
3. sanbaan =						
4. neippalsep =						
5. aptcoenaul =						
6. rebrebslieu =						
7. wabreriestrs =						
8. pergaftuir =						
9. sperag =						
10. yapaap =						
11. twiirfkui =						
12. shercrie =						
13. yhweeond =						
14. sapre =						
15. gantrinsee =						
16. coptairs =						
17. slomen =						
18. tnelwamero =						
19. muslp =						
20. chepsea =						
21. gisf =						
22. dovcaao =						
23. snirrrbeeca =						
24. semli =						
25. acaabs =						

Mixed Fruit

Activity B   Name _____

Chapter 18   Date _____ Period _____

Describe quality factors you should seek when selecting each of the following fruits in its specified form. Explain how to properly store each type of fruit. Then describe how to prepare the fruit for its specified use. If no use is specified, indicate how you would choose to serve the fruit and describe the preparation technique.

1. Fruit: frozen strawberries

     Use: _____

     Selection: _____

     _____

     _____

     Storage: _____

     _____

     _____

Preparation:

_____

_____

_____

_____

_____

_____

2. Fruit: fresh bananas

     Use: fresh fruit salad

     Selection: _____

     _____

     _____

     Storage: _____

     _____

     _____

Preparation:

_____

_____

_____

_____

_____

_____

3. Fruit: canned peaches

     Use: _____

     Selection: _____

     _____

     _____

     Storage: _____

     _____

     _____

Preparation:

_____

_____

_____

_____

_____

_____

4. Fruit: raisins

     Use: cooked raisin sauce

     Selection: _____

     _____

     _____

     Storage: _____

     _____

     _____

Preparation:

_____

_____

_____

_____

_____

_____

Vegetables

Vegetable Selection and Storage

Activity A

Chapter 19

Name_____

Date_____ Period _____

The following statements about selecting and storing vegetables are false. Rewrite them to make them true.

1. Vegetables are often classified according to their size and shape. _____
   _____

2. Broccoli, green peppers, and raw cabbage are excellent sources of protein._____
   _____

3. When selecting vegetables, select those that are very large. _____
   _____

4. Fresh vegetables retain their quality for a long while, so keep large quantities on hand.
   _____
   _____

5. Vegetables that are in season are usually high in quality and, therefore, high in price.
   _____
   _____

6. Vegetables should be soaked in water to remove soil and pesticides before using.
   _____
   _____

7. To save money when buying canned vegetables, choose reduced-price, dented cans.
   _____
   _____

8. Canned vegetables retain the appearance and flavor of fresh vegetables better than frozen and dried
   vegetables. _____
   _____

9. To be sure vegetables are solidly frozen, choose packages with a heavy layer of ice on them.
   _____
   _____

10. Dried vegetables of greatest commercial importance are onions, mushrooms, and potatoes.
    _____   _____
    _____   _____

Vegetable Maze

Activity B   Name _____

Chapter 19   Date _____ Period _____

Complete the statements by writing terms related to vegetables in the blanks. Then find the terms in the word maze and circle them. (Terms are located forward, backward, horizontally, vertically, and diagonally in the maze.)

```
A  I  C  K  A  C  I  A  D  F  H  S  G  E  A  Q  B  F  J  O  V  A  S
N  A  Q  B  L  A  N  C  H  I  N  G  S  L  N  R  S  D  E  E  S  H  S
T  E  V  Y  N  M  A  E  O  R  C  S  K  E  I  O  I  O  U  R  E  Y  N
H  P  G  T  L  R  H  R  P  E  G  A  E  F  P  O  R  H  A  N  T  J  I
O  R  O  E  V  F  E  L  B  U  L  O  S  R  E  T  A  W  N  K  R  U  K
C  A  D  S  T  E  M  N  F  I  E  X  T  E  R  U  G  R  U  K  E  G  S
Y  S  O  K  J  A  D  D  S  Q  M  Z  N  I  H  O  E  M  U  I  X  D  B
A  R  B  Y  A  Z  B  E  E  A  E  M  E  V  A  B  D  Q  H  L  C  B  G
N  E  Q  E  B  E  I  L  R  N  C  E  L  L  U  L  O  S  E  E  W  A  D
I  W  E  S  X  L  P  D  E  U  N  N  U  T  S  L  B  A  R  Y  E  E  N
N  O  A  O  T  S  O  J  U  B  S  A  C  O  N  A  B  L  X  K  N  T  L
W  L  A  N  I  Z  R  D  M  A  R  R  C  T  I  M  Y  F  O  E  A  F  V
E  F  Y  R  Z  C  O  C  L  B  L  U  U  G  E  S  V  W  T  U  F  N  W
U  J  C  K  W  P  L  Z  E  U  P  T  S  C  F  I  U  O  D  W  C  C  H
S  O  S  S  E  N  O  V  A  L  F  U  C  H  L  O  R  O  P  H  Y  L  L
K  U  M  O  I  B  C  L  K  B  O  H  L  I  L  A  E  J  D  S  I  L  M
A  X  O  A  D  O  S  G  N  I  K  A  B  W  C  T  U  O  W  K  E  V  M
```

1. Asparagus and celery come from the _____ part of the plant.

2. A vegetable _____ can be used to remove dirt from the crevices of vegetables.

3. Vegetables with a high moisture content are called _____.

4. _____-_____ nutrients in vegetables, such as vitamin C, B-vitamins, and minerals, can be lost during cooking or soaking.

5. Carrots, radishes, and beets are the _____ part of the plant.

1. _____

2. _____

3. _____

4. _____

5. _____

Name _____

6. Garlic and onion are the _____ part of a plant.

6. _____

7. When vegetables are cooked, the _____ is softened, which makes chewing easier.

7. _____

8. Cooked vegetables should have a _____-tender texture when served.

8. _____

9. Potatoes come from a part of a plant called a _____.

9. _____

10. Red vegetables contain a pigment called _____.

10. _____

11. Peas, corn, and beans are the _____ of plants.

11. _____

12. _____ vegetables usually cost less than either fresh or frozen vegetables.

12. _____

13. _____, the pigment in green vegetables, is sensitive to heat.

13. _____

14. Although _____ _____ will turn chlorophyll a bright green during cooking, it also causes the loss of some important nutrients.

14. _____

15. Deep yellow vegetables contain _____, a source of vitamin A.

15. _____

16. Potatoes that are sent to market immediately after harvesting are called _____ potatoes.

16. _____

17. If there is _____ in the cooking water, red vegetables will turn purple.

17. _____

18. _____ are pigments contained in white vegetables.

18. _____

19. Preheating vegetables in boiling water or steam to prepare them for freezing is known as _____.

19. _____

20. Dried peas and beans must be _____ before cooking.

20. _____

21. A small amount of an _____, such as vinegar or lemon juice, will neutralize alkaline cooking water and prevent vegetables from changing color.

21. _____

22. Besides flavor and the part of the plant, vegetables can be classified by _____.

22. _____

23. Artichokes and broccoli are the _____ of plants.

23. _____

24. Vegetables cooked in their _____ will retain more nutrients.

24. _____

25. Fresh vegetables cost less when purchased during their _____ growing season.

25. _____

Cooking Vegetables by Class

Activity C   Name _____

Chapter 19   Date _____ Period _____

In each of the following items, identify the pigment that gives vegetables the specified color. Describe the cooking method generally recommended for cooking vegetables of that color. Then give an example of a vegetable in that color category.

1. Green pigment: _____

   Cooking method: _____

   _____

   _____

   Example: _____

2. Yellow pigment: _____

   Cooking method: _____

   _____

   _____

   Example: _____

3. White pigment: _____

   Cooking method: _____

   _____

   _____

   Example: _____

4. Red pigment: _____

   Cooking method: _____

   _____

   _____

   Example: _____

Place each of the following vegetables in the appropriate flavor category in the chart below. Then describe the cooking method generally recommended for cooking vegetables in that category.

beets	corn	parsnips
broccoli	green beans	peas
Brussels sprouts	leeks	spinach
cabbage (green)	onions	yellow turnips

5. Mildly Flavored Vegetables	6. Strongly Flavored Vegetables	7. Very Strongly Flavored Vegetables
Cooking method:	Cooking method:	Cooking method:

Salads, Casseroles, and Soups

Salads

Activity A

Chapter 20

Name _____

Date _____ Period _____

Complete the following exercises about salads.

1. Explain why greens should be washed before they are used. _____

_____

_____

2. Why should greens be torn instead of cut with a knife? _____

_____

_____

Match each salad dressing to its description by placing the correct letter in the space provided.

3. A dressing that is a temporary emulsion made by combining oil, vinegar, and seasonings.

4. An uncooked dressing containing egg yolks that is a permanent emulsion.

5. A dressing that is thickened with a food starch and is cooked.

_____ A. cooked salad dressing

_____ B. French salad dressing

_____ C. mayonnaise

6. Give a specific example of each of the following types of salads.

Protein salad: _____

Pasta salad: _____

Vegetable salad: _____

Fruit salad: _____

Gelatin salad: _____

7. Create a salad. List the ingredients to be included in the salad. Then attach a sketch of the salad. Label the base, body, dressing, and the garnish parts of the salad.

Ingredients: _____   _____

_____   _____

_____   _____

_____   _____

Sketch:

Casserole Preparation Guide

Activity B   Name _____

Chapter 20   Date _____ Period _____

List eight items in each of the casserole ingredient categories below. Then answer the questions that follow to provide tips on putting a casserole together.

Protein Foods	Vegetables
A.	A.
B.	B.
C.	C.
D.	D.
E.	E.
F.	F.
G.	G.
H.	H.
Starchy Foods	**Sauces**
A.	A.
B.	B.
C.	C.
D.	D.
E.	E.
F.	F.
G.	G.
H.	H.
Extras	**Toppings**
A.	A.
B.	B.
C.	C.
D.	D.
E.	E.
F.	F.
G.	G.
H.	H.

1. Why do leftover foods work well as casserole ingredients? _____

_____

2. How can cleanup of baked casseroles be made easier? _____

_____

3. How can you keep the topping on a casserole from getting too dark? _____

_____

Stock Soups

Activity C

Chapter 20

Name _____

Date _____ Period _____

Match the following descriptions with the correct terms by placing the correct letter in the blank provided.

_____ 1. The stock resulting when poultry, fish, or unbrowned meat is cooked in a liquid.

_____ 2. The stock resulting when browned meat is cooked in a liquid.

_____ 3. A process done to separate broth from solid materials.

_____ 4. The stock that results when slightly beaten egg white and a few pieces of eggshell are added to a boiling broth.

_____ 5. A clear broth made from stock.

_____ 6. A clear, rich-flavored soup made from stock.

A. bouillon

B. brown stock

C. clarified stock

D. consommé

E. light stock

F. straining

G. unbrowned stock

The steps required for preparing bouillon are listed below. Place the numbers 1 through 10 in the blanks to reorganize the steps in the correct order.

_____ Fat is removed from the surface of the soup.

_____ The stock is strained to remove the egg, solid materials, and eggshell.

_____ The ingredients are placed in a large pan and covered with water.

_____ The pan is covered with a tightly fitted lid and the ingredients are simmered for several hours.

_____ The meat, poultry, fish, and vegetables to be used in the stock are cut into small pieces.

_____ The strained, clarified stock is reduced in volume by further cooking.

_____ The stock is strained to separate the solid materials from the broth.

_____ Foam is skimmed from the surface of the soup.

_____ The stock is clarified.

_____ The meat is browned.

Herbs, Spices, and Blends

Activity D　　　　　Name _____

Chapter 20　　　　　Date _____ Period _____

List the seasonings you have in your foods laboratory. Check the appropriate column to indicate whether each is an herb, a spice, or a blend. Identify the type(s) of food(s) in which each seasoning is used. Then complete the items at the bottom of the page.

Seasoning	Type (✓)			Used to Flavor
	Herb	Spice	Blend	

1. Explain how herbs, spices, and blends differ.

_____

_____

_____

2. Describe how to store herbs, spices, and blends properly.

_____

_____

Cereals

Grains and Grain Products

Activity A

Chapter 21

Name_____

Date _____ Period _____

1. Label and describe the three main parts of this kernel of grain.

A. _____
_____
_____

B. _____
_____
_____

C. _____
_____
_____

Name the most important grains used for food in the United States by unscrambling the letters and writing the correct terms in the blanks.

2. H A T E W   _ _ _ _ _ _

3. R O N C   _ _ _ _

4. L A E Y B R   _ _ _ _ _ _

5. A T O S   _ _ _ _

6. I R E C   _ _ _ _

7. Y R E   _ _ _

Match the following descriptive phrases with the correct terms.

_____ 8. A flour made from a blend of different varieties of wheat that is used for general cooking purposes.

_____ 9. A flour made from soft wheat that is used for cakes and other baked products with delicate textures.

_____10. A flour made from the entire wheat kernel that gives baked products a nutlike flavor and coarse texture.

_____11. Macaroni, noodles, and spaghetti.

_____12. Cereal products to which thiamin, niacin, riboflavin, and iron have been added in specified amounts.

_____13. The seed of a grass that grows in the marshes of Minnesota and Canada.

_____14. Corn minus the hull and germ.

_____15. The refined starch from the endosperm of corn.

_____16. Whole wheat that has been cooked, dried, partly debranned, and cracked.

_____17. A wheat product made by grinding and sifting wheat from which the bran and most of the germ has been removed.

A. all-purpose flour

B. bulgur wheat

C. cake flour

D. cornstarch

E. enriched

F. farina

G. hominy

H. pasta

I. pearl barley

J. whole wheat flour

K. wild rice

Breakfast Cereal Comparison

Activity B   Name _____

Chapter 21   Date _____ Period _____

Record information from the Nutrition Facts labels of your choice of two ready-to-eat breakfast cereals in the spaces provided. Then answer the questions on the next page.

Cereal A:	Cereal B:
Price:	Price:
Servings per container:	Servings per container:
Nutrition information per serving without milk	
Serving size:	Serving size:
Calories:	Calories:
Calories from fat:	Calories from fat:
Total fat:	Total fat:
Saturated fat:	Saturated fat:
Cholesterol:	Cholesterol:
Sodium:	Sodium:
Total carbohydrate:	Total carbohydrate:
Dietary fiber:	Dietary fiber:
Sugars:	Sugars:
Protein:	Protein:
Percent Daily Value	
Total fat:	Total fat:
Saturated fat:	Saturated fat:
Cholesterol:	Cholesterol:
Sodium:	Sodium:
Total carbohydrate:	Total carbohydrate:
Dietary fiber:	Dietary fiber:
Vitamin A:	Vitamin A:
Vitamin C:	Vitamin C:
Calcium:	Calcium:
Iron:	Iron:
Other nutrients:	Other nutrients:
List the first five ingredients shown on the label	

(Continued)

Name _____

1. Which cereal is the most economical? _____

2. Which cereal is lowest in fat? _____

3. Which cereal is lowest in sodium? _____

4. Which cereal is lowest in sugar?_____

5. Which cereal is highest in fiber? _____

6. Which cereal is highest in vitamins and minerals? _____

7. Which cereal would you rank as most nutritious overall? Explain your answer. _____

   _____

   _____

8. Which cereal would you rather eat? Explain your answer. _____

   _____

   _____

9. What size portion of this cereal do you typically eat? _____

10. How does this portion size affect your evaluation of nutrition label information?_____

   _____

   _____

11. What type of milk do you pour on your cereal? _____

12. How does the milk affect the nutritive value of the cereal?_____

   _____

   _____

13. How much, if any, sugar do you add to your cereal before eating it? _____

14. How does added sugar affect the nutritive value of the cereal?_____

   _____

Starch and Cereal Cookery

Activity C   Name_____

Chapter 21   Date _____ Period _____

Read the following statements about starch and cereal cookery. Circle *T* if the statement is true. Circle *F* if the statement is false.

T   F   1. Starch is a simple carbohydrate stored in animals.

T   F   2. Cornstarch- and tapioca-thickened mixtures are opaque.

T   F   3. All starches behave the same way during cooking.

T   F   4. Granular starch is soluble in both hot and cold water.

T   F   5. Dry heat causes starch to lose some of its thickening power.

T   F   6. When starch granules are combined with liquid and heated, they absorb the liquid and swell.

T   F   7. To prevent overcooking, starch mixtures should be removed from the heat as soon as gelatinization occurs.

T   F   8. Gentle stirring during cooking will help keep starch mixtures smooth.

T   F   9. Coating starch granules with fat will prevent lumping.

T   F   10. The relative low cost and high energy value of cereals make them an important part of the diet.

T   F   11. Adding salt to the cooking water for cereals is optional.

T   F   12. Whole grain cereals will cook more quickly if they are first soaked to soften the bran.

T   F   13. Cooking cereals at temperatures that are too hot can cause lumping and scorching.

T   F   14. Cereals that are finely granulated or precooked will cook slower than cracked or whole grain cereals.

T   F   15. Properly cooked rice is tender and fluffy.

T   F   16. White rice, brown rice, and instant rice all cook in about the same amount of time.

T   F   17. As the starch granules swell, pasta doubles in size.

T   F   18. Pasta should be added to cold water.

T   F   19. Pasta products should be rinsed after draining.

T   F   20. When cooked in a microwave oven, rice and cereal should be allowed to stand a few minutes before serving.

Breads

Functions of Ingredients

Activity A   Name_____

Chapter 22   Date _____ Period _____

The principal ingredients used in baked products are pictured below. In the space provided, list at least one function of each of these ingredients in baked products.

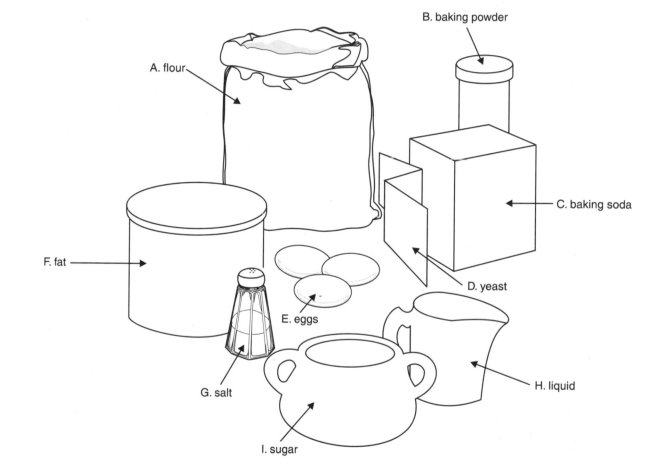

A._____

B._____

C._____

D._____

E._____

F._____

G._____

H._____

I._____

Adjusting Recipes

Activity B   Name _____

Chapter 22   Date _____ Period _____

Rewrite the ingredient list for the recipe below to reflect minimum ingredient proportions.

Old-Fashioned Biscuits (Makes 12 biscuits)	**Light 'n Healthy Biscuits** (Makes 12 biscuits)
2 cups flour	_____
2 teaspoons sugar	_____
1 tablespoon baking powder	_____
1 teaspoon salt	_____
⅓ cup shortening	_____
¾ cup milk	_____

Use the following information to calculate the savings in calories, fat, and sodium that will result from the adjustments you made to the recipe:

• Sugar provides 15 calories per teaspoon.

• Baking powder provides 390 mg of sodium per teaspoon.

• Salt provides 2000 mg of sodium per teaspoon.

• Shortening provides 115 calories and 13 g of fat per tablespoon.

• Skim milk provides 65 calories and 8 g of fat less per cup than whole milk.

Total calorie savings _____

Calorie savings per biscuit _____

Total fat savings _____

Fat savings per biscuit _____

Total sodium savings _____

Sodium savings per biscuit _____

Characteristics of Quick Breads

Activity C   Name_____

Chapter 22   Date _____ Period _____

Answer the following questions about the characteristics of quick breads.

1. What are two differences between rolled biscuits and dropped biscuits?_____

   _____

   _____

   _____

2. Describe the characteristics of a high-quality rolled biscuit. _____

   _____

   _____

   _____

3. Read the characteristics below. Write *O* in the blank if the characteristic describes an overmixed muffin. Write *U* in the blank if the characteristic describes an undermixed muffin. Write *H* in the blank if the characteristic describes a high-quality muffin.

   _____ A. coarse crumb   _____ F. symmetrical top that looks rough

   _____ B. flat top   _____ G. tender, light crumb

   _____ C. low volume   _____ H. thin, evenly browned crust

   _____ D. pale, slick crust   _____ I. tunnels

   _____ E. peaked top   _____ J. uniform texture

4. Why is the oven temperature for popovers changed part way through the baking period?_____

   _____

   _____

   _____

5. What happens to a popover that has not been baked long enough? _____

   _____

6. What can happen to cream puffs if the oven door is opened during baking? _____

   _____

7. What occasionally causes cream puffs to ooze fat during baking?_____

   _____

Yeast Breads

Activity D   Name _____

Chapter 22   Date _____ Period _____

Complete the following exercises dealing with yeast breads.

1. Explain how to knead yeast bread dough. _____

   _____

   _____

   _____

   _____

   _____

2. Why is yeast bread kneaded? _____

   _____

3. Characteristics of yeast breads are listed below. Check those that are signs of a high-quality loaf of yeast bread.

   _____ A. large volume   _____ F. fine and uniform texture

   _____ B. small volume   _____ G. crumbly

   _____ C. smooth, rounded top   _____ H. tender and elastic crumb

   _____ D. sunken top with overhanging sides   _____ I. contains large, overexpanded cells

   _____ E. coarse texture   _____ J. compact texture

4. In the spaces below, sketch two ways yeast bread dough can be shaped.

Cakes, Cookies, Pies, and Candies

Kinds of Cakes

Activity A

Chapter 23

Name _____

Date _____ Period _____

Complete the following exercises about cakes.

1. Check all of the following characteristics that apply to shortened cakes.
   _____ A. They contain fat.
   _____ B. They contain no fat.
   _____ C. Butter cake is an example of a shortened cake.
   _____ D. A sponge cake is an example of a shortened cake.
   _____ E. They are leavened by baking powder or baking soda and sour milk.
   _____ F. They are tender, moist, and velvety.
   _____ G. They come out moist and tasty when prepared in a microwave oven.

2. How do pound cakes differ from other shortened cakes? _____
   _____
   _____

3. Check all of the following characteristics that apply to unshortened cakes.
   _____ A. They are sometimes called *foam cakes*.
   _____ B. They contain no fat.
   _____ C. Angel food cake is an example of an unshortened cake.
   _____ D. Chocolate cakes are unshortened cakes.
   _____ E. They are leavened by air beaten into eggs and by steam formed during baking.
   _____ F. They microwave well.

4. How do sponge cakes differ from other unshortened cakes? _____
   _____
   _____

5. Check all of the following characteristics that apply to chiffon cakes.
   _____ A. They contain fat.
   _____ B. They contain beaten egg whites.
   _____ C. They are a cross between shortened and unshortened cakes.
   _____ D. They contain no eggs or fat.

Match each of the following functions to the basic ingredient that performs it in cakes by placing the correct letter in the corresponding blank.

_____ 6. Gives sweetness to cakes, tenderizes the gluten, and improves the texture of cakes.

_____ 7. Gives structure to a cake.

_____ 8. Causes a cake to rise.

_____ 9. Tenderizes the gluten.

_____ 10. Used in angel food and sponge cakes to make the grain of the cake finer and to stabilize the egg white proteins.

_____ 11. Provides flavoring.

_____ 12. Improves the flavor and color of cakes and helps to leaven some cakes.

_____ 13. Provides moisture.

A. cream of tartar
B. egg
C. fat
D. flour
E. leavening
F. liquid
G. salt
H. sugar
I. vanilla extract

Preparation of Cakes

Activity B   Name _____

Chapter 23   Date _____ Period _____

The statements below describe preparation principles and techniques used in preparing cakes. In the space provided, give a reason for each principle or step.

Principles of Preparation

1. Measure the flour accurately. _____

   _____

2. Avoid overmixing the ingredients. _____

   _____

3. Bake the batter in pans of the correct size. _____

   _____

4. Do not grease pans for unshortened cakes. _____

   _____

5. Bake the cake just until it tests done. _____

   _____

Baking Shortened Cakes

6. Pans should not touch each other or the oven while baking. _____

   _____

7. Insert a wooden toothpick into the center of the cake, or lightly touch the center of the cake with your fingertip. _____

   _____

8. Allow the cake to cool in the pan for about 10 minutes. _____

9. When microwaving shortened cakes, use a round or ring-shaped pan. _____

   _____

Preparing Unshortened Cakes

10. Eggs should be at room temperature. _____

    _____

11. After pouring batter into the pan, run a spatula through the batter. _____

    _____

12. Gently touch the cracks that form in the top of the cake. _____

    _____

13. When the cake is done, place the cake upside down over the neck of a bottle. _____

    _____

Cookies

Activity C   Name _____

Chapter 23   Date _____ Period _____

Various kinds of cookies are given below along with the six basic groups of cookies. Indicate to which group each kind of cookie belongs by writing the corresponding letter in the blank.

A. rolled   D. refrigerator
B. dropped   E. pressed
C. bar   F. molded

_____ 1. spritz   _____ 6. oatmeal cookies

_____ 2. gingerbread   _____ 7. brownies

_____ 3. pinwheel   _____ 8. chocolate chip cookies

_____ 4. sugar cookies   _____ 9. crescents

_____ 5. lemon squares   _____ 10. chocolate ball cookies

Read the following statements about cookies. Circle *T* if the statement is true. Circle *F* if the statement is false.

T   F   11. Cookies are easier to make than cakes.

T   F   12. Rolled cookies are made from a stiff dough.

T   F   13. Dropped cookies do not spread as much as rolled cookies during baking.

T   F   14. Refrigerator cookies contain a high proportion of fat.

T   F   15. Most cookies contain more fat and sugar and less liquid than cakes.

T   F   16. The conventional mixing method used for shortened cakes is used to mix all types of cookies.

T   F   17. Cookie sheets should not have high sides, or cookies will bake unevenly.

T   F   18. Cookie sheets should be hot when cookies are placed on them for baking.

T   F   19. Cookie sheets should touch the sides of the oven when cookies are baking.

T   F   20. Large numbers of dropped cookies can be efficiently prepared in a microwave oven.

T   F   21. Crisp cookies should be stored in a container with a tight-fitting cover.

T   F   22. Many cookies freeze well both in dough form and after baking.

Pie Filling

Activity D   Name _____

Chapter 23   Date _____ Period _____

Supply the requested information about different kinds of pies.

1. Describe a typical fruit pie. _____

2. Describe a typical cream pie.

3. Describe a typical custard pie. _____

4. Describe a typical chiffon pie.

5. Describe the characteristices of a high-quality pie. _____

6. Describe your favorite kind of pie. _____

Pastry Preparation

Activity E

Name _____

Chapter 23

Date _____ Period _____

Answer the following questions about pastry preparation.

1. Check each statement that applies to the steps used in preparing a pastry to be used for a one-crust pie that will be filled after baking.

_____ A. Flour and salt are sifted into a mixing bowl.

_____ B. Flour and salt are spooned and packed into a mixing bowl.

_____ C. Shortening is cut into the flour-salt mixture with a pastry blender.

_____ D. Shortening is melted and added to the flour.

_____ E. The shortening, flour, and salt are cut together until large lumps are formed.

_____ F. The shortening, flour, and salt are cut together until the particles resemble coarse cornmeal.

_____ G. Water is added all at once to the flour mixture.

_____ H. Water is sprinkled a little at a time over the flour mixture.

_____ I. The dough is stirred gently with a fork until it forms large lumps.

_____ J. The dough is kneaded.

_____ K. The dough is gathered and gently pressed into a ball.

_____ L. The dough is rolled out on an unfloured surface.

_____ M. The dough is rolled out on a floured surface.

_____ N. The dough is rolled out in a circle about ⅛ inch (3 mm) thick and 1 inch (2.5 cm) larger than the pie plate.

_____ O. The dough is stretched to fit the pie plate.

_____ P. The dough is folded and gently fitted into the pie plate.

_____ Q. The edges of the pie crust are fluted, and the bottom and sides are pricked.

_____ R. The crust is baked for 8 to 10 minutes until it is lightly browned.

_____ S. The crust is baked for 20 to 25 minutes until it is crispy.

2. How would the above preparation steps differ if the pastry was to be filled before baking?

_____

_____

3. How would the above preparation steps differ if the pastry was to be used for a two-crust pie?

_____

_____

4. How would the above preparation steps differ if the pastry was to be prepared in a microwave oven?

_____

Candy

Activity F

Chapter 23

Name _____

Date _____ Period _____

Read the clues below. Write C in the blank if the clue describes crystalline candy. Write NC in the blank if the clue describes noncrystalline candy. If the clue describes both types of candy, write B in the blank.

_____ 1. Fudge is an example.

_____ 2. Caramels are an example.

_____ 3. Peanut brittle is an example.

_____ 4. Divinity is an example.

_____ 5. Toffee is an example.

_____ 6. Fondant is an example.

_____ 7. A sugar syrup is used.

_____ 8. The sugar syrup is heated to a specific temperature, cooled to a specific temperature, and beaten vigorously.

_____ 9. The sugar syrup is heated to a very high temperature.

_____10. Substances like corn syrup, milk, cream, or butter are added to interfere with crystallization.

_____11. A candy thermometer is used for accuracy.

_____12. The use of a heavy saucepan is recommended.

_____13. For best results, the recipe must be followed exactly.

_____14. The sugar syrup forms small, fine crystals.

_____15. The sugar syrup does not form crystals.

16. What is a sugar syrup and what does it have to do with candy making? _____

_____

17. Describe high-quality fudge. _____

_____

18. Describe high-quality peanut brittle. _____

_____

19. What is the advantage of using a microwave oven to melt chocolate, caramels, and marshmallows for use in recipes? _____

_____

20. What, if any, type of candy can be made in a microwave oven? _____

Parties, Picnics, and Dining Out

Planning a Party

Activity A

Chapter 24

Name _____

Date _____ Period _____

Choose a party theme. Complete the invitation below with the date, time, place, and any other information about the party that your guests will need to know. Then complete the party planning activities that follow.

> ## *You Are Invited To:*
> *What?* _____
> *When?* _____
> *Where?* _____
> *R.S.V.P.* _____

In the space provided, plan a menu of familiar recipes for the party described in the invitation. Be sure to list only items for which you have all the needed equipment.

_____   _____

_____   _____

_____   _____

_____   _____

Describe how you will serve the refreshments or meal you have planned.

_____

_____

What is your budget for the party? $ _____

How much will you have to spend for the food items listed in the menu above?   – _____

How much will you have left to spend on decorations and entertainment? $ _____

(Continued)

115

116   *Guide to Good Food*

Name _____

Put a star by each of the items in the menu on the previous page that you can prepare in advance. In the space below, plan a time schedule for preparing the remaining menu items on the day of the party.

Time	Tasks

How will you decorate for this party?

_____
_____
_____

How will you and your guests dress for this party?

_____
_____
_____

Make a list of what you need to do to get ready for this party besides preparing food.

_____
_____
_____

Describe three planned activities that are good ways to break the ice at parties.

1. _____
_____
2. _____
_____
3. _____
_____

List three responsibilities of a good guest.

1. _____
2. _____
3. _____

Table Manners

Activity B   Name _____

Chapter 24   Date _____ Period _____

Solve each situation below by providing an appropriate solution.

1. You sit down at the table. What do you do with your napkin?

    1. _____
    _____
    _____

2. Bread is served with the meal. How do you eat it?

    2. _____
    _____
    _____

3. You are eating with your right hand. What do you do with your left hand?

    3. _____
    _____
    _____

4. You have an olive pit in your mouth. How do you get it out?

    4. _____
    _____
    _____

5. The salad dressing you would like is across the table. How do you get it?

    5. _____
    _____
    _____

6. There are three forks next to your plate. How do you know which one to use first?

    6. _____
    _____
    _____

7. You have dropped an eating utensil. What do you do?

    7. _____
    _____
    _____

8. You start to have a sneezing spell. What do you do?

    8. _____
    _____
    _____

9. A food to which you are allergic has been served. What do you do?

    9. _____
    _____
    _____

10. You have just finished eating. What do you do with the flatware?

    10. _____
    _____
    _____

Food and Beverages for Parties

Activity C   Name _____

Chapter 24   Date _____ Period _____

Complete the following descriptions of a hot appetizer and a cold appetizer you could make ahead to serve for a party. Be sure your choices reflect variety in flavors, colors, and textures.

Hot Appetizer	**Cold Appetizer**
Name of recipe: _____	Name of recipe: _____
Ingredients: _____	Ingredients: _____
_____	_____
_____	_____
_____	_____
_____	_____
_____	_____
Appearance/Color: _____	Appearance/Color: _____
_____	_____
Texture: _____	Texture: _____
_____	_____

Read the clues below. If the clue describes coffee, write *C* in the blank. If the clue describes tea, write *T* in the blank. If the clue describes hot chocolate or cocoa, write *HC* in the blank. If the clue described a cold drink, write *CD* in the blank.

_____ 1. This beverage is made from the leaves of a small tropical evergreen.

_____ 2. This beverage is made from seeds of the cocao tree.

_____ 3. This beverage is often served in a punch bowl.

_____ 4. Depending on the preparation method, this beverage might be made from medium or coarse grind.

_____ 5. This beverage is made from special beans that are dried and roasted.

_____ 6. This beverage can be prepared using the syrup method or the paste method.

_____ 7. The three main types are black, green, and oolong.

_____ 8. This beverage may be made in a percolator.

_____ 9. This beverage may be served with a straw.

_____10. Because milk and sugar are used to prepare this beverage, low temperatures must be used to prevent scorching.

Entertaining Outdoors

Activity D

Chapter 24

Name_____

Date_____ Period _____

Suggest a menu that would be appropriate for a picnic or a barbecue.

_____

_____

_____

_____

_____

_____

_____

_____

Place a check next to each statement that describes a safe barbecuing technique.

_____ 1. Always place the grill in the open, away from trees, shrubbery, furniture, and buildings.

_____ 2. Use gasoline to start the fire.

_____ 3. Wear loose-fitting clothes.

_____ 4. If you have long hair, tie it back away from your face.

_____ 5. Once the fire has started, never pour more lighter fluid over the coals.

_____ 6. Place the grill in an enclosed area.

_____ 7. Keep all flammable materials, such as lighter fluid, away from the fire.

_____ 8. Keep a container of water handy.

Make a list of items to pack in a picnic basket.

_____   _____

_____   _____

_____   _____

_____   _____

_____   _____

_____   _____

_____   _____

_____   _____

_____   _____

_____   _____

_____   _____

Dining Out

Activity E

Chapter 24

Name _____

Date _____ Period _____

Give the name of a restaurant in your area for each of the types of restaurants shown in the chart below. Then complete the chart with information about the specific restaurants you listed. You may wish to use the entertainment section of a newspaper or metropolitan magazine or a local dining guide to help you complete this activity.

Type of Restaurant	Atmosphere	Menu Items Available	Price Range	Popular Characteristics
Fast food				
Cafeteria/Buffet				
Family restaurant				
Formal restaurant				
Specialty restaurant				

In which of the above restaurants do you prefer to eat? Explain your answer.

_____

_____

_____

_____

Preserving Foods

Microorganisms and Enzymes

Activity A   Name _____

Chapter 25   Date _____ Period _____

Read the following phrases. If the phrase describes microorganisms, circle *M*. If the phrase describes enzymes, circle *E*. Then answer the questions below.

M   E   1. They include bacteria, mold, and yeast.

M   E   2. They are complex proteins produced by living cells.

M   E   3. They are used in making buttermilk and sauerkraut.

M   E   4. They are used in curing some cheeses such as Roquefort and Camembert.

M   E   5. They ripen foods.

M   E   6. They tenderize meats.

M   E   7. Their action is controlled most often by extreme temperatures.

M   E   8. They need food, moisture, and favorable temperatures to grow.

M   E   9. Their growth is prevented by freezing temperatures.

M   E   10. Their action is retarded by freezing temperatures.

11. Describe how freezing temperatures affect microorganisms and enzymes. _____

_____

_____

_____

12. Describe how high temperatures, such as those used in canning, affect microorganisms and enzymes. _____

_____

_____

_____

13. Describe how drying prevents the growth of microorganisms. _____

_____

_____

_____

14. Describe how enzyme activity can be controlled in dried fruits and vegetables. _____

_____

_____

_____

Home Canning

Activity B   Name _____

Chapter 25   Date _____ Period _____

Select the answer that best completes each of the following statements and write the letter in the blank.

_____ 1. Most foods are canned at home in _____.
   A. glass jars
   B. aluminum cans

_____ 2. A flat metal lid for a home canning jar should be _____.
   A. reused
   B. used only once

_____ 3. Pressure canning is used for _____ foods.
   A. low-acid
   B. high-acid

_____ 4. In a pressure canner, steam is released through the _____.
   A. pressure gauge
   B. petcock

_____ 5. In boiling water canning, processing time begins when _____.
   A. the canner is placed on the heat
   B. the water comes to a rolling boil

_____ 6. Boiling water canning would be suitable for _____.
   A. green beans
   B. peaches

_____ 7. Open kettle canning, oven canning, and steam canning are _____.
   A. safe for many foods
   B. not recommended canning methods

_____ 8. When canning jars are completely cool, screw bands are _____.
   A. carefully removed
   B. left on for storage

_____ 9. If a leaky jar is found, canned food should be _____.
   A. discarded
   B. used right away

_____10. Home-canned foods should be stored in a _____ place.
   A. cool, dry, dark
   B. cool, moist, dark

Read the following statements about checking for spoilage in home-canned foods. If the statement is true, circle *T*. If the statement is false, circle *F*.

T   F   11. If you believe a home-canned food is spoiled, taste it to be certain.

T   F   12. Flat-sour spoilage can be caused by a delay in processing or failure to cool jars quickly.

T   F   13. Always heat low-acid canned foods before eating them.

T   F   14. If a food looks spoiled, foams, or has an off odor, destroy it.

T   F   15. Some spoiled foods may look and smell normal.

T   F   16. Botulism is the most dangerous type of food spoilage.

T   F   17. Bulging lids and leaks are signs of broken seals and spoilage.

T   F   18. Home-canned foods with broken seals are safe to eat.

Jellied Products Crossword

Activity C

Chapter 25

Name _____

Date _____ Period _____

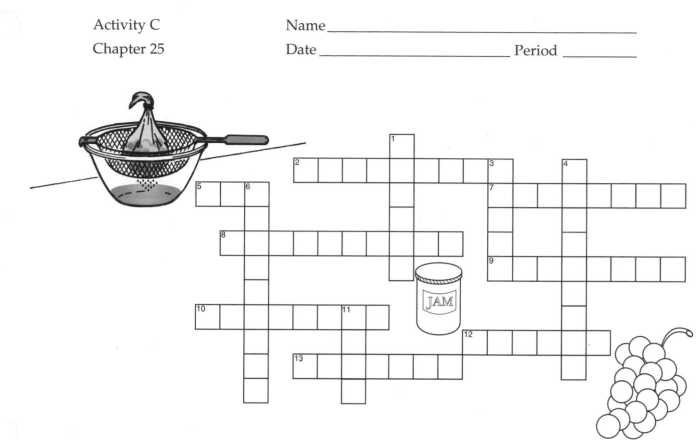

Across

2. Slightly jellied whole or large pieces of fruit are called _____.
5. Crushed fruit cooked to a fairly even consistency is used to make _____.
7. _____ jams keep up to three weeks in the refrigerator, but they spoil quickly at room temperature.
8. _____ _____ is the basic ingredient that gives jelly its flavor and color.
9. The pectin and acid content of fruits are greatly affected by _____.
10. Juice is extracted from fruit with the aid of a _____ _____.
12. Fruit _____ is made from cooked, pureed fruit, but it is not a jellied product.
13. Jellies should be processed in a _____ water canner.

Down

1. Unripe fruits have more _____ than mature, ripe fruits.
3. _____ helps jelly become firm.
4. Raisins and nuts are sometimes added to _____.
6. _____ is a tender jelly often made from citrus fruits.
11. _____ works along with pectin to make fruit juices jell.

Freezing

Activity D   Name_____

Chapter 25   Date _____ Period _____

Complete the following statements about freezing food. Then arrange the circled letters to spell a term related to freezing food. Answer the questions that follow.

1. When a food is _ __O__ _-_ _ _ _ _ _ _, it is subjected to an extremely low temperature of –25° to –40°F (–32° to –40°C) for a short time and then maintained at a normal freezing temperature of 0°F (–18°C).

2. If food is frozen slowly, large _ _ _ _ _ _O_ _ _ _ form that damage the cell structure of the food and change its texture.

3. The main piece of equipment required to freeze food is a _ _ _O_ _ _ _.

4. Dry, tough areas that occur where dry air from the freezer comes in contact with food surfaces are called _ _ _ _ _ _ _ _ _O_.

5. _ _ _O_ _ _ _ _ _ made of plastic, glass, aluminum, and plastic-coated paper are suitable for storing frozen foods.

6. _ _ _ _ _ _ _O_ _ fruits may develop a bitter or off flavor during freezing.

7. Frozen fruits are often treated with _ _ _ _O_ _ _ acid to preserve color and flavor and to add nutritive value.

8. When packing foods to be frozen, 1 inch (2.5 cm) of _ _O_ _ _ space should be left to allow for expansion.

9. Thawing fruits in their original covered container will prevent discoloration caused by exposure to air, which is called _ _ _ _ _O_ _ _ _ _ _ _ _ _ _ _ _.

10. Most vegetables must be _ _ _O_ _ _ _ before freezing to inactivate enzymes that can cause spoilage.

11. When freezing meats, you may wish to trim large cuts and package them in appropriate _ _ _O_ _ _-sized pieces.

12. Containers used in freezing must be moisture- and _ _ _O _-resistant to protect food from exposure to air and loss of moisture.

Circled letters: _____

Freezing is one method of food _ _ _ _ _ _ _ _ _ _ _ _ _.

13. How should frozen fruits be served?_____

_____

14. How should frozen meat, poultry, and fish be thawed?_____

_____

15. How do you determine when partially thawed food can be refrozen? _____

Drying

Activity E   Name _____

Chapter 25   Date _____ Period _____

The steps for preparing, sun drying, and storing fruits and vegetables are listed below. Reorganize the steps so that they are in the correct order. Then answer the questions that follow.

Steps:

1. _____   A. Allow vegetables to become dry and brittle and fruits to become leathery and pliable.
2. _____   B. Blanch vegetables and sulfur fruits.
3. _____   C. Cover tray with a piece of cheesecloth.
4. _____   D. Cut fruits and vegetables into pieces that will dry quickly and evenly.
5. _____   E. Occasionally stir food to ensure even drying.
6. _____   F. Package dried foods in insectproof and moistureproof containers.
7. _____   G. Place tray in direct sunlight.
8. _____   H. Seal and label containers.
9. _____   I. Select young, tender vegetables in prime condition and fruits at optimum maturity.
10. _____ J. Spread food in a single layer on drying tray.
11. _____ K. Store containers in a cool, dark place.
12. _____ L. Wash fruits and vegetables.

13. Briefly explain how drying preserves food. _____

_____

14. List five examples of commercially dried food products. _____

_____

15. Why are dried foods popular with campers, hikers, and backpackers? _____

_____

16. Describe a treatment other than sulfuring that can be used to keep fruit from darkening. _____

_____

17. Why do trays with screen bottoms allow foods to dry faster than cookie sheets?_____

_____

18. What two appliances can be used to oven dry foods? _____

19. How are dried vegetables prepared for cooking? _____

_____

20. How long can dried fruits and vegetables be stored on a shelf?_____

Storage Life of Foods

Activity F
Chapter 25

Name _____

Date _____ Period _____

Give the storage life for each food listed below according to the type of storage indicated.

Freezer

1. Beef _____
2. Bread _____
3. Fish _____
4. Frozen
   vegetables _____
5. Ground
   meat _____
6. Hot dogs _____
7. Ice cream _____
8. Lamb _____
9. Pork _____
10. Poultry _____

Refrigerator

11. Bacon _____
12. Beef _____
13. Natural
    cheese _____
14. Fish _____
15. Fruit _____
16. Pork _____
17. Poultry _____
18. Vegetables _____

Shelf

19. Aseptically
    packaged
    juice _____
20. Canned
    peaches _____
21. Dried beans _____
22. Flour _____
23. Home-canned
    tomatoes _____
24. Onions _____
25. Raisins

Regional Cuisine of the United States

Cultural Influences on Food

Activity A

Chapter 26

Name _____

Date _____ Period _____

Color in a region on the map below. Then answer the questions regarding food customs in that region.

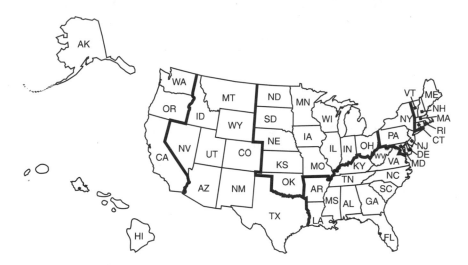

Region: _____

1. What group(s) of people settled this region? _____

2. What foods are native to this region? _____
   _____

3. How did the settlers use these native foods to prepare the dishes of their homeland(s)? _____
   _____

4. What foods were introduced by the settlers? _____
   _____

5. What cooking methods were used by the settlers? _____
   _____

6. How did cultural customs and traditions affect the types of foods and cooking methods used by the settlers? _____
   _____

7. What dishes introduced by the settlers are still typical of this region today? _____
   _____

8. How do dishes typically served in this region today reflect the culture of the people who settled the region? _____
   _____

U.S. Regions Maze

Activity B

Chapter 26

Name _____

Date _____ Period _____

Complete the statements by writing terms related to regional cuisines of the United States in the blanks. Then find the terms in the word maze and circle them. (Terms are located forward, backward, horizontally, vertically, and diagonally in the maze.)

```
C E P L M T E K S A B D A E R B L C R S
A L O E R T Y L F O O H S Z T T S I K E
X P A W O A U E O B S Y F O I E N M B L
V A A M N A S D G E R U I T H X S M A Y
A M C O C S N Z K H R Z H Y D X W I R O
Q N R K C H R S E R U C I G J J F G S W
E A T B J H O C F G T Y U E I V T R F K
U V N B L U H W J U L J A M B A L A Y A
H I N I L E G Q D D G V N A U E H N W U
G B U F C O N I L E V I T A N U M T J A
U L O M I P O E Y B R I T I S H M S Q V
O O K B O L L E F N T P U O I W I U T L
D C R D L D E I U Q O N X G U M U R U Z
R E A P Z A M J L T E M R A P R M L U X
U K T A S G A P L E R S U O H O I P T K
O D F U N C G U M B O L Q N M S O S Y U
S T S A O C C I F I C A P X Z S T A M I
J A E O Q K H I N S R V E N E W R U O Y
```

1. Food customs in the United States began with the _____ Americans, who settled in organized groups, or tribes.

2. The first permanent colonists in the United States were the _____, who established settlements in Jamestown and Plymouth.

3. Groups of _____ from various European countries settled together in particular regions of the United States.

4. Many people associate New England with _____ _____, which is a creamy soup made with potatoes and clams.

5. New Englanders boiled down sap from trees to make _____ syrup.

6. A group of German immigrants who settled in the southeast section of Pennsylvania were the Pennsylvania _____.

1. _____

2. _____

3. _____

4. _____

5. _____

6. _____

(Continued)

Name _____

7. A Pennsylvania Dutch pastry with a filling made of molasses and brown sugar is _____ pie.

7. _____

8. Food customs of African slaves are combined with food customs of Native Americans and European sharecroppers in _____ _____.

8. _____

9. A green, pod-shaped vegetable that was brought to the United States from Africa is _____.

9. _____

10. Sweet potatoes that have moist, orange flesh are _____.

10. _____

11. Cooking techniques of the French and ingredients of the Africans, Caribbeans, Spanish, and Native Americans are combined in _____ cuisine.

11. _____

12. A flavoring and thickening agent made from sassafras leaves is _____.

12. _____

13. A soup that reflects the various cultures of Southern Louisiana is _____.

13. _____

14. A traditional Creole dish that contains rice; seasonings; and shellfish, poultry, and/or sausage is _____.

14. _____

15. The hearty fare of rural Southern Louisiana is called _____ cuisine.

15. _____

16. People often call the agriculturally productive Midwest the _____ of the nation.

16. _____

17. A shared meal to which each person or family brings food for the whole group to eat is called a(n) _____.

17. _____

18. Wild _____ animals, such as antelope, rabbit, and deer, account for much of the meat eaten in remote areas of the West.

18. _____

19. The cattle introduced in the West and Southwest by the Spanish eventually developed into the _____ breed.

19. _____

20. California, Oregon, Washington, and Alaska form the _____ _____ region.

20. _____

21. A dough containing active yeast plants that was used as a leavening agent by gold prospectors is _____.

21. _____

22. Christian missionaries who came to Hawaii in the early 1800s introduced a loose garment called a(n) _____.

22. _____

23. Hawaii's three largest industries are pineapple, sugarcane, and _____.

23. _____

24. An elaborate outdoor feast that is popular in the Hawaiian Islands is a(n) _____.

24. _____

25. A rock-lined pit used to roast a whole pig at a Hawaiian feast is called a(n) _____.

25. _____

Regional Foods Match

Activity C   Name _____

Chapter 26   Date _____ Period _____

Match the following regions of the United States with the foods typical of each region. (There are three matches for each region.)

_____ _____ _____   1. New England

_____ _____ _____   2. Mid-Atlantic

_____ _____ _____   3. South

_____ _____ _____   4. Midwest

_____ _____ _____   5. West and Southwest

_____ _____ _____   6. Pacific Coast

_____ _____ _____   7. Hawaiian Islands

A. sopapillas
B. andouille
C. sourdough bread
D. barbecued beef
     short ribs
E. caribou sausage
F. coconut
G. shoofly pie
H. whole wheat
     bread
I. succotash
J. poi
K. macadamia nuts
L. baked beans
M. jambalaya
N. scrapple
O. chitterlings
P. apple pie
Q. broiled steak
R. clam chowder
S. salmon steaks
T. chicken corn soup
U. tamales

List the groups of people that influenced the cuisines in each region of the United States.

New England: _____

Mid-Atlantic: _____

South: _____

Midwest: _____

West and Southwest: _____

Pacific Coast: _____

Hawaiian Islands: _____

Latin America

Chapter **27**

Mexican Cuisine

Activity A

Chapter 27

Name _____

Date _____ Period _____

The foods listed below are all important in Mexican cuisine. For each item, if the food was contributed by the Aztecs, write *A* in the blank. If the food was contributed by the Spanish, write *S* in the blank. Then answer the questions that follow.

_____ 1. peppers

_____ 2. chicken

_____ 3. wheat

_____ 4. chocolate

_____ 5. wine

_____ 6. corn

_____ 7. vanilla

_____ 8. pineapples

_____ 9. rice

_____ 10. beans

_____ 11. tomatoes

_____ 12. beef

_____ 13. cinnamon

_____ 14. oil

_____ 15. squash

_____ 16. avocados

17. Name three staple ingredients in Mexican cuisine. Describe a dish made with each of the ingredients.

    A. _____

    B. _____

    C. _____

18. List three vegetables and three fruits grown in Mexico. Describe one Mexican fruit or vegetable dish.

    Vegetables: _____

    Fruits: _____

    Fruit or vegetable dish: _____

19. Identify two different regions of Mexico and describe a dish typical of each region.

    A. _____

    B. _____

20. Name two meals served in Mexico and describe foods typically served at those meals.

    A. _____

    _____

    B. _____

    _____

Latin America Maze

Activity B   Name _____

Chapter 27   Date _____ Period _____

Complete the statements by writing terms related to Latin America in the blanks. Then find the terms in the word maze and circle them. (Terms are located forward, backward, horizontally, vertically, and diagonally in the maze.)

```
S  A  N  A  N  A  B  A  A  S  N  B  O  U  T  Y  P  W  E  A
O  R  O  D  A  P  S  A  D  A  N  A  P  M  E  J  Q  F  N  E
Z  E  T  E  U  T  Z  Y  Y  I  T  O  R  T  I  L  L  A  M  J
I  B  O  N  I  S  O  W  U  Q  D  T  I  V  I  E  V  C  A  C
T  A  M  A  L  E  S  R  C  H  I  L  E  A  N  S  J  Z  N  X
S  I  D  P  P  G  U  A  C  A  M  O  L  E  E  Y  T  Y  I  M
E  U  P  C  L  M  D  E  A  U  E  B  O  J  S  E  A  E  O  U
M  N  A  R  L  A  A  H  U  D  X  B  R  Y  C  X  C  A  C  S
O  Y  V  Q  A  P  N  E  Z  E  I  I  E  S  L  I  O  W  L  A
L  A  A  P  H  B  H  T  S  G  C  Y  M  B  R  W  I  U  I  P
I  S  S  E  O  M  R  E  A  R  O  O  E  H  I  X  L  R  V  M
N  N  S  P  K  D  Q  B  F  I  H  S  M  E  I  A  R  A  B  A
I  R  A  P  M  T  E  T  A  F  N  M  S  I  F  F  O  G  O  P
L  N  C  E  Y  A  T  E  T  G  A  S  L  A  D  F  Q  E  N  R
L  N  S  R  N  R  G  H  L  U  L  L  X  U  Z  A  O  T  W  K
O  F  H  S  I  N  A  P  S  V  F  U  H  A  G  P  A  C  N  I
```

1. The Latin American country that is located closest to the United States is _____.

2. The _____, who controlled Mexico until the middle of the nine-teenth century, greatly influenced Mexican culture, especially in architecture, language, and food customs.

3. When _____ was introduced to Mexican cuisine, it enabled many foods to be fried in deep fat or on lightly greased griddles.

4. People of mixed European and Native American ancestry, who are called _____, make up the largest percentage of Mexico's population.

5. _____ are a staple food in Mexico used to make frijoles refritos.

6. Over 30 varieties of _____ are used in Mexican cuisine.

7. Mashed avocado, tomato, onion, and spices are used in Mexico to make a spread called _____.

8. The _____ are the richest lands in South America and reach into the countries of Argentina and Uruguay.

9. Argentine appetizers that are small turnovers filled with chopped meat, olives, raisins, and onions are called _____.

1. _____

2. _____

3. _____

4. _____

5. _____

6. _____

7. _____

8. _____

9. _____

(Continued)

Name _____

10. Of all the South Americans, _____ probably eat the most seafood.

10. _____

11. In some regions, manioc is known as _____.

11. _____

12. _____ are green, starchy fruits that have a bland flavor and look much like large bananas.

12. _____

13. Colombian _____ trees thrive on the cool slopes of the Andes Mountains.

13. _____

14. _____ are made by stuffing small amounts of corn dough with meat and beans and tucking them into corn husks and roasting them.

14. _____

15. A popular Afro-Brazilian coconut pudding contains _____, a Brazilian staple food.

15. _____

16. The Brazilian version of the Mexican tamale, called _____, is a mixture of cowpeas, shrimp, pepper, and dendé oil rolled into banana leaves and cooked over an open fire.

16. _____

17. Because Ecuador is a large producer of _____, they are featured in many local snacks, desserts, and breads.

17. _____

18. The original inhabitants of Mexico were the _____.

18. _____

19. In Mexico, the main meal of the day is called _____.

19. _____

20. A _____ is a flat, unleavened bread made from cornmeal and water that is used to make many Mexican dishes.

20. _____

21. A _____ is a crisp, fried tortilla filled with meat, beans, shredded lettuce, and cheese and seasoned with chili.

21. _____

22. A starchy root plant eaten as a side dish and used in flour form in cooking and baking throughout South America is _____.

22. _____

23. Mexican chocolate is beaten into a frothy foam with the aid of a tool called a _____.

23. _____

24. The _____ were a group of Native South Americans who built a large empire in the Andes Mountains.

24. _____

25. _____ is a caramel custard served as a Mexican dessert.

25. _____

South American Culture and Cuisine

Activity C   Name _____

Chapter 27   Date _____ Period _____

Identify each of the South American countries indicated on the map. Match each food listed below with the country to which it is most associated. Then provide a brief description of how the food is served or used.

ajiaco   dendé oil

arepa   papa

bananas   pastel de choclo

chimichurri

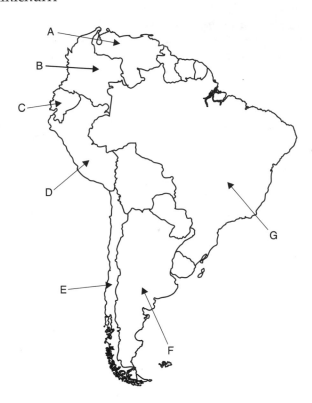

A.   Country: _____

     Food: _____

     _____

B.   Country: _____

     Food: _____

     _____

C.   Country: _____

     Food: _____

     _____

D.   Country: _____

     Food: _____

     _____

E.   Country: _____

     Food: _____

     _____

F.   Country: _____

     Food: _____

     _____

G.   Country: _____

     Food: _____

     _____

Europe

British Food and Customs

Activity A

Chapter 28

Name _____

Date _____ Period _____

1. Label the four countries indicated on the map of the British Isles.

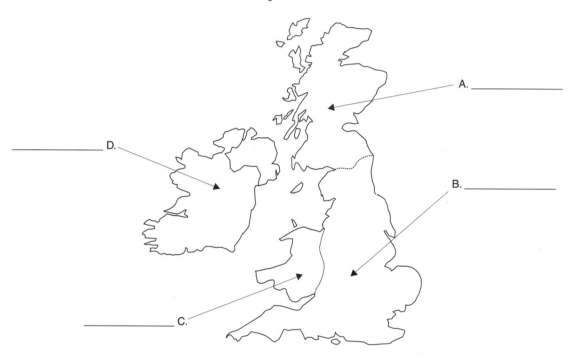

A. _____

D. _____

B. _____

C. _____

Match the countries in the map with each of the following phrases about British food and customs. Place the letter of the country that is most closely associated with each phrase in the blank.

_____ 2. Hogmanay

_____ 3. toad in the hole

_____ 4. House of Lords

_____ 5. cockles

_____ 6. cawl

_____ 7. potatoes

_____ 8. kilts

_____ 9. finnan haddie

_____ 10. fish and chips

_____ 11. coal mines

_____ 12. Buckingham Palace

_____ 13. soda bread

_____ 14. St. Patrick's Day

_____ 15. peat burned for heat and cooking

_____ 16. bagpipes

_____ 17. Welsh rabbit

_____ 18. cock-a-leekie

_____ 19. steamed puddings

_____ 20. crempog

_____ 21. pink-colored pearl

_____ 22. corned beef and cabbage

_____ 23. haggis

_____ 24. bubble and squeak

_____ 25. the small green island

France Crossword

Activity B

Chapter 28

Name _____

Date _____ Period _____

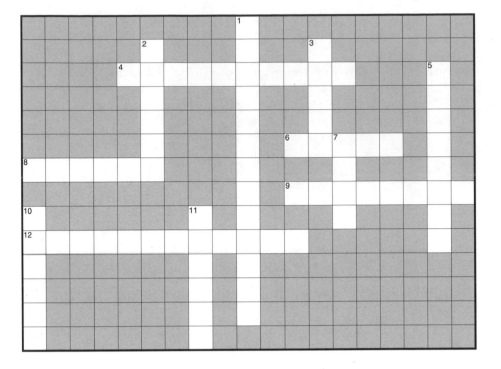

Across

4. Locally grown foods and simple cooking methods are used in _____ cuisine, which is the style of cooking practiced by most French families.
6. _____, such as chives, parsley, tarragon, and chervil, are often used to flavor French soups and stews.
8. Escargots are _____ eaten as food and are a specialty of Burgundy.
9. _____ cuisine is a style of French cooking that emphasizes lightness and natural taste in foods.
12. Small dishes designed to stimulate the appetite are called _____.

Down

1. _____ is the leading industry in France.
2. Favorable climatic conditions in France encourage the growth of _____, which are used to make wine.
3. _____ cuisine is a style of French cooking characterized by elaborate preparations, fancy garnishes, and rich sauces.
5. _____, a rare type of fungi that grow underground near oak trees, are harvested by people who use pigs to sniff the ground to find them.
7. A _____ is a mixture of butter (or other fat) and flour that forms the base of white sauces used in French cooking.
10. Fresh fruit and _____ are often served after the green salad and before the sweet dessert in a large French meal.
11. A custard tart, known as a _____, originated in Lorraine.

Foods of Germany

Name_____

Date_____ Period_____

Complete the following statements about German foods by filling in the blanks using the words below.

kasseler rippenspeer	Westphalian ham	spätzle
sauerbraten	braunschweiger	pumpernickel
hasenpfeffer	bratwurst	strudel
preiselbeeren	kartoffelpuffer	lebkuchen
schnitzel	sauerkraut	stollen
salzkartoffeln	eintopf	gebildbrote

1. _____ is a sausage made of freshly ground, seasoned pork that is usually cooked by grilling.

2. Small dumplings made from wheat flour called _____ are a popular German side dish.

3. _____ is a rabbit dish that is braised in a marinade of wine, vinegar, onions, and spices.

4. Small, cranberry-like fruits called _____ are often served with game dishes.

5. _____ is a richly flavored, smoked uncooked ham that is served throughout Germany.

6. Young men and women sometimes give the honey-spice cake called _____ to their sweethearts as gifts.

7. _____ is a whole smoked pork loin that is roasted and served with sauerkraut, apples or chestnuts, peas, white beans, mushrooms, and browned potatoes.

8. _____ is fermented or pickled cabbage that is usually flavored with caraway, apple, onion, or juniper berries and served with pork dishes.

9. _____ is a type of liver sausage that was first produced in Braunschweig, Germany.

10. _____ is a breaded, sautéed veal cutlet.

11. At Christmastime, Germans may serve a rich yeast bread called _____, which is filled with almonds, raisins, and candied fruit.

12. _____ bread, made from unsifted rye flour, is a favorite in Germany.

13. _____, a sweet-sour marinated beef roast, is a popular beef dish in Germany.

14. A German dessert made with paper-thin layers of pastry filled with plums, apples, cherries, or poppy seeds is called _____.

15. _____ are the famous potato pancakes enjoyed throughout Germany.

16. Breads baked into fanciful shapes are called _____, which means picture breads.

17. _____ are potatoes cooked in salted water that are drained and steamed until dry.

18. Leftovers are used to make _____, a popular stew.

Influences on Scandinavian Cuisine

Activity D   Name _____

Chapter 28   Date _____ Period _____

Use complete sentences to answer the following questions about Scandinavian climate, geography, and cuisine.

1. A. Briefly describe the seasonal climate of Norway, Sweden, and Finland. _____

_____

   B. How has climate affected food production in these countries? _____

_____

   C. How has climate affected food preparation in these countries?_____

_____

2. A. Briefly describe the geography of Norway, Sweden, and Finland. _____

_____

   B. How has geography affected food production in these countries? _____

_____

3. How does Denmark's climate differ from that of the other Scandinavian countries?_____

_____

4. How does Denmark's geography differ from that of the other Scandinavian countries? _____

_____

5. How do climate and geography affect food production in Denmark? _____

_____

_____

6. What industry is important to all four Scandinavian countries? _____

_____

7. What are Denmark's main agricultural products? _____

_____

8. What are the main agricultural products of the other Scandinavian countries? _____

_____

9. How does Danish cuisine differ from that of the other Scandinavian countries? _____

_____

_____

10. Give an example with a brief description of a dish typical of each of the Scandinavian countries.

   A. Denmark: _____

   B. Norway: _____

   C. Sweden: _____

   D. Finland:_____

Cuisine Travel Guide

Activity E

Chapter 28

Name_____

Date _____ Period _____

Pretend you are a travel agent. Part of your job involves designing travel brochures for a "Cuisines of Europe" travel package being offered by your company. On these pages, design a travel brochure for one of the European countries. Provide some background on the country and then focus on the cuisine so that people will want to visit the country. Place drawings or pictures from newspapers or magazines in the boxes to illustrate your brochure. Use your creativity to develop a descriptive, interesting brochure rather than just a fact sheet.

Country:_____

Climate _____

_____

_____

Geography _____

_____

_____

Size: _____

Capital city: _____

General Information

Population:_____

Language spoken:_____

Historical background:_____

_____

_____

_____

_____

Form of government: _____

Primary religion: _____

Major industries: _____

_____

_____

_____

(Continued)

Name _____

Customs and beliefs: _____
_____

Native costume: _____

Holidays: _____

Points of interest: _____

Cuisine
Common ingredients: _____
_____

Typical dishes (list five, describe two): _____
_____
_____
_____

Characteristics of the cuisine: _____
_____
_____

Preparation methods: _____
_____

Meal patterns: _____
_____

Serving customs: _____
_____

Mediterranean Countries   Chapter 29

Spanish Culture and Cuisine

Activity A

Chapter 29

Name _____

Date _____ Period _____

Match the following descriptions related to the culture and cuisine of Spain with the terms they describe. Place the correct letter in the corresponding blank.

_____ 1. Some people call this country the "land of romance."

_____ 2. This large plateau occupies more than half of Spain.

_____ 3. This group of people established colonies in Spain along the Mediterranean coast as early as 1100 B.C.

_____ 4. Many Spaniards make their living in these industries.

_____ 5. This is a Spanish omelet.

_____ 6. This is one of the most popular pastimes in Spain.

_____ 7. This term, which means food of the people, describes Spanish cuisine.

_____ 8. The Romans contributed these ingredients to Spanish cuisine.

_____ 9. These people crossed into Spain from Africa in A.D. 711, bringing many cultural and culinary advances.

_____ 10. Spanish cooking should not be confused with the spicy cooking of this country.

_____ 11. Vegetables, beef, lamb, ham, poultry, and a spicy sausage cook together in a large pot to make this dish.

_____ 12. This is a fish soup in which all the ingredients are cooked together for 15 minutes.

_____ 13. This soup is often made with coarsely pureed tomatoes, onions, garlic, and green peppers; olive oil; and vinegar.

_____ 14. This Spanish rice dish has many variations.

_____ 15. This wine-based punch is served throughout Spain.

_____ 16. These are Spanish appetizers.

_____ 17. This perfumed type of wine is popular in Spain.

_____ 18. This fleet of armed ships was defeated in 1588.

_____ 19. This garlic mayonnaise is served with seafood in some parts of Spain.

_____ 20. This dark sausage has a spicy, smoky flavor.

_____ 21. This Spanish sauce is flavored and colored with large amounts of parsley.

_____ 22. These grilled foods are served as appetizers.

_____ 23. This second morning meal is served at around 11 o'clock.

_____ 24. The Spanish use this term to refer to dried beans, lentils, and chick-peas.

_____ 25. These small pieces of vegetables, meat, poultry, or fish are battered, deep-fried, and served as appetizers.

A. all-i-oli

B. almuerzo

C. banderillas

D. bullfight

E. buñuelitos

F. chorizo

G. cocido

H. del pueblo

I. fishing and farming

J. gazpacho

K. Meseta

L. Mexico

M. Moors

N. olive oil and garlic

O. paella

P. Phoenicians

Q. pinchos

R. pulses

S. salsa verde

T. sangria

U. sherry

V. sopa al cuarto de hora

W. Spain

X. Spanish Armada

Y. tapas

Z. tortilla

Italian Foods Identification

Activity B   Name _____

Chapter 29   Date _____ Period _____

Identify each of the following Italian foods. Write *S* in the blank if the food is a type of seafood. Write *H* in the blank if the food is an herb. Write *P* in the blank if the food is a type of pasta. Write *C* in the blank if the food is a cheese. Then answer the questions that follow.

_____ 1. Parmesan   _____ 13. marjoram

_____ 2. orecchietta   _____ 14. cannelloni

_____ 3. fusilli   _____ 15. Romano

_____ 4. tarragon   _____ 16. ricotta

_____ 5. mozzarella   _____ 17. spaghetti

_____ 6. sardines   _____ 18. anchovies

_____ 7. oregano   _____ 19. provolone

_____ 8. sole   _____ 20. parsley

_____ 9. ricci di donna   _____ 21. thyme

_____ 10. sage   _____ 22. gorgonzola

_____ 11. mussels   _____ 23. squid

_____ 12. oysters   _____ 24. lasagne

25. A. How do the pastas served in Northern Italy differ from those served in Southern Italy? _____

_____

_____

_____

_____

B. Describe a dish that is a specialty of Northern Italy. _____

_____

_____

C. Describe a dish that is a specialty of Southern Italy. _____

_____

_____

Italian Culture and Cuisine

Activity C

Chapter 29

Name _____

Date _____ Period _____

Read the following statements about Italian culture and cuisine. Circle *T* if the statement is true. Circle *F* is the statement is false.

T   F   1. During the Renaissance period, Italian cooking became the "mother cuisine"—the source of all other western cuisines.

T   F   2. The most productive farming area in Italy is the Po River Valley, which is located in the northern part of the country.

T   F   3. Rome, Italy's capital city, is located in Northern Italy.

T   F   4. The Greeks colonized Sicily and Southern Italy.

T   F   5. The powerful Roman Empire is credited with achievements in art, architecture, law, and government.

T   F   6. Almost all Italians are Roman Catholics.

T   F   7. Southern Italy is the richest part of the country in natural resources.

T   F   8. The beginning of Italian cuisine belongs to the Greeks.

T   F   9. Italy laid the foundation for French haute cuisine.

T   F   10. Italian cooks rely heavily on convenience foods.

T   F   11. Many Italian foods are baked or roasted in the oven.

T   F   12. Pasta, a paste made from wheat flour that is dried in various shapes, is eaten throughout Italy.

T   F   13. Pasta should be served al dente, or slightly resistant to the bite.

T   F   14. Because of the vast coastline of Italy, seafood is one of the Italian staple foods.

T   F   15. The Italians introduced ice cream to the rest of Europe.

T   F   16. Italian foods are bland because herbs and spices are seldom used.

T   F   17. Wine often replaces water at Italian meals.

T   F   18. Culinary divisions occur between Northern Italy and Southern Italy.

T   F   19. Southern Italian cooking is the cooking with which most people in the United States are familiar.

T   F   20. Northern Italian foods are spicy.

T   F   21. A Northern Italian specialty is pollo alla cacciatore.

T   F   22. Spaghetti is seldom served in Rome.

T   F   23. Cheesecake was invented by the Romans.

T   F   24. Southern Italian dishes feature rich tomato sauces.

T   F   25. Antipasto is the dessert course of an Italian meal.

Greece Maze

Activity D   Name _____

Chapter 29   Date _____ Period _____

Complete the statements by writing terms related to the culture and cuisine of Greece in the blanks. Then find the terms in the word maze and circle them. (Terms are located forward, backward, horizontally, vertically, and diagonally in the maze.)

```
S G Y L D O O F A E S S E S L L S Y O
A B F N Z E J B P K C O R T H O D O X
H A A K A S S U O M S E G G P L A N T
H E R B S O D O D E R K G N R I M F L
O S A W E I B C H T L A C I S S A L C
N N S R D K T D N A E O I P U Y U O I
E E U L O D E E A V W N L P H I Z X T
Y H B O M Z I B F E A P M I W H N K Y
C T C B E C Q E C R T T A H V V F T S
E A A M N Z N O F N N E T S D E E M T
A Y F A R M E R S A T U R J T I S W A
O U X L T P B S R S Y G A A U S U G T
A V A L K A B O L L Y H P Q P O L Q E
R Y B O U Z O U K I A I S I R H V N S
```

1. Ancient Greece is sometimes called _____ Greece.   1. _____
2. Ancient Greece was divided into small units called _____ _____.   2. _____
3. _____ was an Ancient Greek city state characterized by a strict, military life governed by stern laws.   3. _____
4. The history of _____ Greece is marked by achievements in art, literature, science, and philosophy.   4. _____
5. The majority of Greeks belong to the Greek _____ Church.   5. _____
6. Although only a small part of the land is suitable for agriculture, a great many Greeks work as _____.   6. _____
7. Many of the wealthiest citizens of Greece are involved in the industry of _____.   7. _____
8. In small Greek communities, people often socialize in cafés called _____.   8. _____

(Continued)

Name _____

9. Greeks often drink _____, a strong, anise-flavored liqueur, when they gather in the evenings at outdoor cafés.

9. _____

10. While gathered at outdoor cafés, Greeks may listen to the sound of a mandolin-like instrument called a _____.

10. _____

11. _____ is the largest city and the capital of Greece.

11. _____

12. Hesiod, a Greek, wrote one of the first _____.

12. _____

13. _____, which are pieces of meat, poultry, fish, vegetables, or fruits threaded onto skewers and broiled, are popular in Greece.

13. _____

14. Many Greek dishes feature _____ and spices, such as basil, cinnamon, dill, bay leaves, oregano, and mint.

14. _____

15. _____ is a fleshy, oval-shaped vegetable with a deep purple skin that is used to prepare the main dish called *moussaka*.

15. _____

16. _____ is a layered main dish containing sliced eggplant, ground lamb, cheese, and a rich cream sauce.

16. _____

17. _____, a meat basic to Greek cooking, may be roasted, broiled, served in casseroles, or added to soups and stews.

17. _____

18. Because Greece is surrounded on three sides by water, _____ is an important part of the Greek diet.

18. _____

19. _____ is a popular type of seafood that is stuffed with rice, onions, nuts, and seasonings; poached; and served as a favorite main dish.

19. _____

20. _____, which grow abundantly in Greece, are eaten as appetizers and snacks or added to other dishes.

20. _____

21. _____ is a slightly salty, crumbly, white cheese made from goat's milk.

21. _____

22. _____, widely used throughout Greek history, is the basic sweetener used in the preparation of many Greek desserts and sweets.

22. _____

23. Greeks make many of their desserts with a paper-thin pastry called _____.

23. _____

24. A popular Greek dessert called _____ is made of phyllo filled with nuts and soaked in a honey syrup.

24. _____

25. In the early evening, Greeks often snack on appetizers called _____.

25. _____

Mediterranean Climate, Geography, and Cuisine

Activity E　　　　　　　Name_____

Chapter 29　　　　　　　Date _____ Period _____

Complete the chart below by briefly describing the climate, geography, and cuisine of each of the Mediterranean countries. Then answer the question that follows.

Country	Climate	Geography	Cuisine
Spain			
Italy			
Greece			

What similarities exist among the three countries?

Climate: _____

Geography: _____

Cuisine:_____

Middle East and Africa

Middle East Match

Activity A

Chapter 30

Name _____

Date _____ Period _____

Match the following descriptions related to the culture and cuisine of the Middle East with the terms that they describe by writing the correct letters in the corresponding blanks.

A. Angora	H. green pepper	O. olive oil
B. bread	I. irrigation	P. Persian
C. coffee	J. Judaism and Islam	Q. rice
D. dolmas	K. lemon	R. spices and herbs
E. eggplant	L. Middle Easteners	S. tea
F. Egypt	M. Nile, Tigris, Euphrates	T. tomato
G. garlic	N. oil	

_____ 1. These fruits and vegetables are basic to all Middle Eastern cooking.

_____

_____

_____

_____

_____ 2. This is an essential means of watering the dry lands of the Middle East.

_____ 3. This country has one of the world's oldest civilizations.

_____ 4. This empire created rugs, tapestries, metalwork, and architecture.

_____ 5. These people make their living as farmers or herders.

_____ 6. This is a type of goat found in Turkey that is the source of mohair fibers.

_____ 7. This is the major natural resource of the Middle East.

_____ 8. These famous rivers are located in the Middle East.

_____ 9. Followers of these religions are forbidden to eat the meat of swine.

_____ 10. This dish contains a mixture of ground meat and seasonings wrapped in grape leaves or stuffed into vegetables.

_____ 11. This ingredient is used in place of butter or lard for cooking.

_____ 12. If this product is dropped on the floor, it must be picked up and kissed.

_____ 13. These are used to give a delicate flavor to foods.

_____ 14. With the exception of Iran, this beverage is served throughout the Middle East.

_____ 15. This is the main beverage of Iran.

Middle East Regional Cuisine

Activity B   Name _____

Chapter 30   Date _____ Period _____

Answer the following questions about similarities and distinctions among the regional cuisines of the Middle East.

1. What food is forbidden by religions widely practiced in all Middle Eastern countries? _____
   _____

2. What is the staple meat in the Middle East? _____

3. What dairy product is served throughout the Middle East in a variety of dishes? _____
   _____

4. What are the staple grains in the Middle East? _____

5. What are the staple legumes in the Middle East? _____

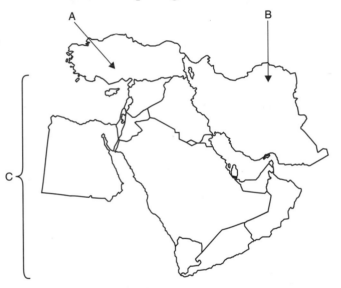

6. Identify each of the Middle Eastern countries indicated on the map.
   A. _____
   B. _____
   C. (Group of countries) _____

Match the countries in the map with each of the following Middle Eastern foods. Place the letter of the country that is most closely associated with each food in the blank.

_____ 7. halva

_____ 8. shrak

_____ 9. torshi

_____ 10. tea

_____ 11. kibbi

_____ 12. chelo

_____ 13. cacik

_____ 14. arak

_____ 15. rahat lokum

_____ 16. döner kebab

_____ 17. khoresh

_____ 18. mazza

_____ 19. khave

_____ 20. hummus

_____ 21. tabbouleh

_____ 22. kurabiye

_____ 23. caviar

_____ 24. polo

Israeli Culture and Cuisine

Activity C   Name _____

Chapter 30   Date _____ Period _____

Read the following statements about the culture and cuisine of Israel. Circle *T* if the statement is true. Circle *F* if the statement is false.

T	F	1.	The land on which Israel is established used to be called *Palestine.*
T	F	2.	Lack of rainfall during the summer months makes irrigation necessary for the production of most crops in Israel.
T	F	3.	Israel imports most of the fruits and vegetables consumed there.
T	F	4.	Many of the farms in Israel operate as collective communities called *kibbutzim.*
T	F	5.	Members of a kibbutz receive wages for their work.
T	F	6.	Jerusalem is called the "Holy City" by Christians, Jews, and Muslims.
T	F	7.	Jewish cuisine is multinational.
T	F	8.	Jewish dietary laws known as *kashrut* are observed in most Israeli homes and restaurants.
T	F	9.	Foods that are not prepared according to Jewish dietary laws are considered to be kosher.
T	F	10.	According to Jewish dietary laws, foods such as shellfish, swine, and wild fowl cannot be consumed.
T	F	11.	According to Jewish dietary laws, all animals and fowl must be slaughtered by a licensed slaughterer known as a *shohet.*
T	F	12.	Milchig and fleishig foods are frequently cooked together to carefully blend the flavors.
T	F	13.	Pareve foods include dairy foods and meats.
T	F	14.	Gefilte is a popular chicken dish.
T	F	15.	Homemade noodles and dumplings are frequent additions to soups, main dishes, and puddings.
T	F	16.	Kugels may be served as side dishes or desserts, depending on the ingredients.
T	F	17.	Tzimmes are combinations of meats, vegetables, and fruits that are quickly fried for a fresh, light flavor.
T	F	18.	Blintzes are layered, torte-like cakes filled with whipped cream.
T	F	19.	Knishes are a type of fish.
T	F	20.	Matzo meal, made from unleavened bread, is used to make knaidlach, mandlen, and latkes.
T	F	21.	Challah is a rich, egg bread that is usually braided and served at Jewish holiday meals.
T	F	22.	Felafel, a mixture of ground chick-peas, bulgur, and spices that is formed into balls and deep-fried, has become one of Israel's national dishes.
T	F	23.	An Israeli delicacy known as leben is a type of cheese made from sour milk.
T	F	24.	Couscous is an Israeli dish with Russian origins.
T	F	25.	Sabra, an Israeli liqueur that has the flavor of the Jaffa orange, is often used to make rich desserts.

An African Buffet

Activity D   Name _____

Chapter 30   Date _____ Period _____

Listed below are foods that are available in Africa. Place an *A* next to the food items that are available in your area.

_____ palm oil	_____ plantains	_____ lamb
_____ groundnuts	_____ chocolate	_____ papaya
_____ bananas	_____ citrus fruits	_____ guava
_____ dates	_____ coffee	_____ cassava
_____ figs	_____ pita bread	_____ okra

Research African recipes. In the space below, write a menu for an African buffet that you might serve to celebrate Kwanzaa. Be sure your menu items include some of the foods listed above that are available in your area.

Menu

_____

_____

_____

_____

_____

_____

Briefly describe how you would arrange the buffet.

_____

_____

_____

_____

In the space below, write a menu for an everyday African meal. Again, be sure your menu items include some of the foods listed above.

Menu

_____

_____

_____

_____

_____

How would this everyday meal be eaten in Africa?

_____

_____

_____

Asia

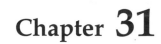

Russian Culture and Cuisine

Activity A

Chapter 31

Name _____

Date _____ Period _____

Complete the following statements about Russian culture and cuisine by using the words below to fill in the blanks.

beef stroganov	blini	Bolsheviks
borscht	caviar	chicken Kiev
czar	kasha	kisel
koumys	kulich	ouba
paskha	pirozhki	samovar
schi	shashlik	zakuska

1. In 1547, Ivan the Terrible became the first _____, or ruler, of Russia.

2. In 1917, Vladimir Lenin led a revolutionary group, called the _____, that took control of the Russian government.

3. A special piece of equipment used to make Russian tea is the _____.

4. A staple food of Russian peasants was _____, which was made from raw grain that was fried and then simmered until tender.

5. Russian appetizers are called _____.

6. A food made from processed, salted eggs of large fish is called _____.

7. Cabbage soup called _____ is one of the most popular Russian soups.

8. Russians often top _____, their well-known beet soup, with a dollop of sour cream.

9. A clear fish broth called _____ is popular in Russia.

10. Cubes of marinated lamb grilled on skewers is a dish called _____, which was developed in the Russian region of Georgia.

11. Tender strips of beef, mushrooms, and a seasoned sour cream sauce are used to make _____.

12. Pounded chicken breasts are wrapped around pieces of butter to make _____, a Russian dish that is popular in the United States.

13. Pancakes made from buckwheat flour, which are called _____, are served as a Russian side dish.

14. _____ are pastries filled with protein-based or sweet fillings.

15. Sour mare's milk, or _____, is one of several dairy products that are important in Russian cooking.

16. Pureed fruit, called _____, was a dessert eaten by Russian peasants.

17. A rich cheesecake molded into a pyramid and decorated with the letters *XB* is the Russian Easter dessert called _____.

18. _____ is a tall, cylindrical yeast cake filled with fruits and nuts that is served as part of the Easter celebration of the Russian Orthodox Church.

Indian Culture and Cuisine

Activity B   Name _____

Chapter 31   Date _____ Period _____

Read the following statements about the culture and cuisine of India. Circle *T* if the statement is true. Circle *F* if the statement is false.

T   F   1. India is the seventh largest country in the world.

T   F   2. In India, the soil in the Ganges River basin is poor and produces only one small crop yield each year.

T   F   3. Foreign invasions, lasting many centuries, contributed to the variety of racial strains and more than 700 different languages and dialects in India today.

T   F   4. English is the official language in India.

T   F   5. The social system known as the caste system developed from Hinduism.

T   F   6. People in India usually cook indoors.

T   F   7. Rice is the major crop grown in India.

T   F   8. In order to feed the vast population in India, large quantities of grain must be imported.

T   F   9. Cattle are raised in India primarily for meat.

T   F   10. The spinning and weaving of wool from India's large sheep herds is India's most important industry.

T   F   11. India's cuisine is not influenced by climate and geography.

T   F   12. The foods of Northern India are hotter than the foods of Southern India.

T   F   13. In Northern India where wheat grows, bread sometimes takes the place of rice at meals.

T   F   14. Religion has been a major influence on the development of Indian cuisine.

T   F   15. Hindus do not eat beef because the cow is considered sacred.

T   F   16. Most Hindus are vegetarians.

T   F   17. Muslims cannot eat pork.

T   F   18. Curry is a sweet made from semolina.

T   F   19. India's coastline provides a variety of fish, which are dried, marinated, and smoked.

T   F   20. Most Indian meat dishes are made with mutton.

T   F   21. Many Indian dishes are cooked in ghee (clarified butter).

T   F   22. Indian cooks use only a few spices in cooking.

T   F   23. Chutneys are mixtures of spices used to make curries.

T   F   24. Indians make many of their sweets from milk.

T   F   25. A tandoor is a clay oven often used in Northern India.

T   F   26. Korma is a cooking technique in which foods are braised, usually in yogurt.

T   F   27. Vinegar and spices create the hot, slightly sour flavor in foods prepared using the vindaloo technique of cooking.

T   F   28. Chasnidarth is an Indian version of the Chinese sweet and sour.

T   F   29. At Indian meals, dishes are served one at a time in special courses.

T   F   30. At Indian meals, diners help themselves to the food by using their fingers.

China Match

Activity C   Name_____

Chapter 31   Date _____ Period _____

Match the following descriptions related to the culture and cuisine of China with the terms they describe. Place the correct letters in the corresponding blanks.

_____ 1. Historically, most of China's people have crowded within this geographic region.

_____ 2. Most modern Chinese people belong to this group, which is a mixture of Mongoloid peoples.

_____ 3. This began when China was unified under the Ch'in Dynasty in 221 B.C.

_____ 4. This last group of foreign invaders arrived in China in the seventeenth century and ruled until the Chinese Republic was declared in 1912.

_____ 5. When the Chinese Communists gained control in 1949, they gave the country this name.

_____ 6. This is China's chief agricultural product.

_____ 7. These are China's most important industrial products.

_____ 8. This versatile Chinese cooking utensil looks like a metal bowl.

_____ 9. This piece of Chinese cooking equipment looks like a round, shallow basket with openings.

_____10. This common Chinese ingredient is a gelatinous, cream-colored cake made from soybeans.

_____11. In this common Chinese cooking method, foods are cooked over high heat in a small amount of fat.

_____12. This well-known Chinese roasted dish is rolled inside thin pancakes with scallions and hoisin sauce.

_____13. This type of noodle is made from flour and eggs and resembles spaghetti.

_____14. This mixture of deep-fried pork cubes, pineapple, and vegetables is served in a sweet-sour sauce.

_____15. This is the Chinese version of an omelet.

_____16. This popular Chinese dessert consists of cubes of almond-flavored gelatin garnished with fruit.

_____17. The Chinese use this term for black tea because black is an unlucky color.

_____18. This thick porridge made from rice or barley is often served for breakfast in China.

_____19. The Chinese enjoy these steamed dumplings filled with meat, fish, vegetables, or sweet fruit as a snack.

_____20. The Chinese use these eating utensils for all dishes except soup and finger foods.

A. almond float

B. bean curd

C. chemicals, porcelain products, and cotton and silk fabrics

D. Chinese Empire

E. Chinese spatula

F. chopsticks

G. congee

H. dim sum

I. Eastern China

J. egg foo yung

K. Han

L. lo mein

M. Manchus

N. Peking Duck

O. People's Republic of China

P. red tea

Q. rice

R. steamer

S. stir-frying

T. sweet and sour pork

U. wok

Japan Maze

Activity D   Name _____

Chapter 31   Date _____ Period _____

Complete the statements by writing terms related to the culture and cuisine of Japan in the blanks. Then find the terms in the word maze and circle them. (Terms are located forward, backward, horizontally, vertically, and diagonally in the maze.)

```
S A P P A R I A R J O S E L T R L K A
A S P W S A I N I J H R Q J F L I G M
E U H G Z U Y X E J T E M P U R A K T
V K D T O C P M Y D D E P K H R M Z S
H I B A C H I S E Q G N X I S M P O O
O Y A A C A A E O I S N O O H P Y T S
E A G B I R W N T F B O W T J B Y L R
R K C E D A I U Z N K X D H E N Q L B
U I T F E I W D T P L U M A U F C O N
A T J S N K E O F I E S N I I P Q S L
S A U E T K A E H H U H V E R K R G A
F B B G A V L S L S O O S H I B O R I
N V S O L N D M D R N Y G O U T E N E
W X S U S E S C T O F U G U F I N I D
E A K E S I A K N T T V A S U R L R H
V I M A H B E I M A O N T A B D I A C
C H R D Y N L U N T Z L E I G U S D P
K S D Z E N O R I C W J E E O T H N Z
X U A W E A C F U I K A Y I R E T A N
B S Q K X D L E Y D P O R Y S G I M Q
```

1. The Japanese work _____ means "clean, light, and sparkling with honesty" and describes the Japanese people, their country, and their cuisine.

2. A _____ is a severe storm that brings heavy rain and damaging winds to Japan during September.

3. In the sixteenth century, the Portuguese were the first _____, or Westerners, to arrive in japan.

4. At the end of World War I, the Japanese government became a military _____.

5. Japan's leading religion is _____, which was introduced by the Chinese.

6. The Japanese word for meal is _____, which means rice.

1. _____

2. _____

3. _____

4. _____

5. _____

6. _____

(Continued)

Name _____

7. _____ is Japanese rice wine.

8. A legume with seeds that are rich in protein and oil is the _____.

9. A custardlike cake made from soybeans is _____.

10. _____, Japanese soy sauce, is an all-purpose seasoning in Japanese kitchens.

11. A Japanese delicacy is blowfish, or _____.

12. Balls of cooked rice flavored with vinegar and served with strips of raw or cooked fish, eggs, vegetables, or seaweed are called _____.

13. A basic Japanese ingredient is _____, which they harvest from surrounding oceans and use both fresh and dried.

14. _____ is a giant white radish, which is a traditional Japanese vegetable.

15. One of the best-known oranges is the mikan, or _____ orange.

16. Japanese cooks prepare _____ by coating vegetables, meat, poultry, and seafood in a batter and quickly frying the coated pieces in oil.

17. Beef _____, which is popular in the United States, is slices of beef glazed with a special sauce.

18. A popular Japanese dish made of thinly sliced meat, bean curd, and vegetables cooked in a sauce is _____.

19. A small grill that can be built into the center of a table or used free standing is a _____.

20. The Japanese serve _____ teas, which are made from unfermented tea leaves.

21. A delicate meal served after the Japanese tea ceremony is _____.

22. Instead of napkins, the Japanese use a small, soft towel called an _____.

23. Umeboshi is a tiny, red _____, which is a traditional Japanese breakfast food.

24. For breakfast, the Japanese often sprinkle rice with a type of dried seaweed called _____.

25. *Tsukemono* is the Japanese term for _____ foods, which are always served at the main meal of the day.

7. _____

8. _____

9. _____

10. _____

11. _____

12. _____

13. _____

14. _____

15. _____

16. _____

17. _____

18. _____

19. _____

20. _____

21. _____

22. _____

23. _____

24. _____

25. _____

Chinese and Japanese Cuisine

Activity E   Name _____

Chapter 31   Date _____ Period _____

The following statements relate to basic ingredients, cooking methods, utensils, serving customs, and meal patterns that are part of Chinese and Japanese cuisine. If a statement relates to Chinese cuisine, write *C* in the blank. If a statement relates to Japanese cuisine, write *J* in the blank. If a statement relates to both Chinese and Japanese cuisines, write *B* in the blank. Then answer the questions that follow.

_____ 1. Sweet desserts are reserved for special occasions.

_____ 2. Aesthetic appearance is an important element of the cuisine.

_____ 3. A cleaver is used to perform all cutting tasks when preparing food.

_____ 4. Fish is more important to the diet than meat.

_____ 5. Three meals are typically served each day.

_____ 6. Soup is eaten with tiny spoons.

_____ 7. A traditional ceremony is performed when tea is served.

_____ 8. Diners show appreciation for the cook's skill by smacking their lips or making sucking sounds.

_____ 9. Five spice powder is an important seasoning.

_____ 10. Foods are eaten with chopsticks.

_____ 11. Steaming is one of the main cooking methods.

_____ 12. A small, soft towel called an *oshibori* is used instead of a napkin.

_____ 13. The wok is used as a versatile cooking utensil.

_____ 14. Foods are cooked on a hibachi.

_____ 15. Tea is the national drink.

_____ 16. Rice is a basic ingredient.

_____ 17. Broiling is a common cooking method.

_____ 18. Stir-frying is the most common cooking method.

19. What similarities exist between the cuisines of China and Japan?

_____

_____

20. What characteristics make Chinese cuisine distinct?

_____

_____

21. What characteristics make Japanese cuisine distinct?

_____

_____